BACK IN THE GAME

WHY CONCUSSION DOESN'T HAVE TO END YOUR ATHLETIC CAREER

BY

JEFFREY S. KUTCHER, MD

WITH

JOANNE C. GERSTNER

OXFORD
UNIVERSITY PRESS

OXFORD
UNIVERSITY PRESS

Oxford University Press is a department of the University of Oxford. It furthers
the University's objective of excellence in research, scholarship, and education
by publishing worldwide. Oxford is a registered trade mark of Oxford University
Press in the UK and certain other countries.

Published in the United States of America by Oxford University Press
198 Madison Avenue, New York, NY 10016, United States of America.

Library of Congress Cataloging-in-Publication Data
Names: Kutcher, Jeffrey S., author. | Gerstner, Joanne C., author.
Title: Back in the game : why concussion doesn't have to end your athletic career / by
Jeffrey S. Kutcher M.D. with Joanne C. Gerstner.
Description: Oxford; New York: Oxford University Press, [2017] | Includes bibliographical
references and index.
Identifiers: LCCN 2015051024 | ISBN 9780190226602 (alk. paper)
Subjects: LCSH: Brain—Concussion—Popular works. | Brain—Wounds and injuries—
Popular works. | Sports injuries in children.
Classification: LCC RC394.C7 K88 2016 | DDC 617.1/027—dc23 LC record
available at http://lccn.loc.gov/2015051024

1 3 5 7 9 8 6 4 2

Printed by Sheridan Books, Inc., United States of America

Like many physicians, I learn something from my patients every single day. It is an honor and privilege to help you heal, stay healthy, and get the most out of life. I am continually inspired by your stories, your sacrifices, and your humanity. This book is dedicated to each and every one of you, as well as the patients I have yet to meet.

I consider myself extremely lucky to have the opportunity to do what I do. Of course, I wouldn't be here without the immense support of my family and friends. I will be forever grateful.

I would like to single out two individuals who provided me with opportunities at the critical early stage of my sports neurology career. Athletic trainer Steve Nordwall invited me onto a football sideline for the first time, completely changing my professional life. Dan Hendrickson, MD, provided support and opened doors along the way with humility and grace.

—*Jeff Kutcher, MD*

My journey into learning about concussions in sports developed in an unexpected way: I found I was writing more and more about them in the late 2000s as a journalist contributing content for the New York Times sports section.

My path, thanks to a Knight–Wallace fellowship at the University of Michigan, led me to Dr. Jeff Kutcher. I became immersed in concussions and sports neurology, trying to observe and learn as much as possible. Dr. Kutcher and his colleagues are at the forefront of the field of sports concussion. They were also unwaveringly open and generous with their time, and they found amazing ways to make neurology—not exactly a simple subject—accessible and understandable to the average person. I am a changed journalist and medical consumer, for the better, from my time at Michigan.

This book is dedicated to the kids who love to play sports, the parents who support them, and the thousands of youth coaches who give their time to touch lives.
—Joanne C. Gerstner

CONTENTS

My entire life has been surrounded by sports—the one thing that can universally bring different cultures, people, religions, and governments together. I grew up playing football, and it has given me so much to be thankful for in life.

In high school, football brought my family together every Friday night. Football provided me with an education at the University of Minnesota and a chance to play in the Big Ten and the highest level of Division I. Football fulfilled a childhood dream of stepping onto an NFL playing field, when I was part of the Indianapolis Colts. That, in turn, led to catching passes from future Hall of Fame quarterback Peyton Manning and winning the 2006 Super Bowl.

But football has also potentially given me other things, such as a future with brain disease, because I sustained multiple concussions during my journey in the game.

Those are the cold, hard facts.

As a husband, and now the father of four beautiful young girls who may also soon step onto an athletic field, I fear a future with possible long-term effects from multiple concussions.

The truth is that concussions are an externality of sports.

They are woven into the fabric of the games we participate in and love to watch. The ever-present reality of concussions in youth sports is why we need to keep discussing this issue.

The talking, however, must be centered—to borrow a famous phrase—on the whole truth and nothing but the truth. Parents, coaches, teachers, athletic directors, and athletes must be informed of the full spectrum of what a concussion is and how it can affect your life in the short and long term.

And there is no better person to take the lead on this issue than trusted neurologist Dr. Jeff Kutcher. As an expert on the brain, Dr. Kutcher has dedicated his life to researching the concussion crisis. But importantly, Dr. Kutcher is even more into delivering personal care for patients dealing with the consequences of concussions and mild traumatic brain injuries. He loves sports and wants to see them flourish. He has a strong desire for sports to take brain health more seriously.

Dr. Kutcher is working toward making the brain a top priority in athletics . . . and he is the type of neurological leader that I am ready to follow!

This book should be the launching pad that helps educate this generation of parents, youth athletes, and coaches, and begins to change the nature of sports.

Let's make our memories matter!

Ben Utecht
2006 Super Bowl Champion, Indianapolis Colts
All–Big Ten Tight End, University of Minnesota

First off, thank you for taking the time to read this. This book is for you, whether you play sports and have been diagnosed with a concussion, you love somebody who has suffered with one, or you just want to learn more about this issue that now appears to be everywhere.

I will start by telling you that I have dedicated my life to improving the neurological health of athletes at all levels. My own journey began when I realized early in my career as a neurologist specializing in treating athletes that while sports-related head trauma can certainly be serious, telling athletes they can no longer play their sports is a very serious proposition as well.

I saw a lot of neurological injury occurring in athletes, and not a lot of concern about it. Caring for athletes with neurological conditions of all kinds requires knowledge, training, critical thinking, and a comprehensive approach.

It does not mean running to the spotlight, commercializing a product, or hiring a public relations firm. I care about my patients and their neurological health, completely and without distraction. I do not let the "wide world of sports" cloud my focus, whether I'm on the sideline, in my clinic, or in the academic arena.

The thing is, the brain and neurological health are extremely complicated subjects.

At a basic level, we seem to understand that sports are good. They get our kids moving, engaging them in dynamic ways and providing a means for them to grow and mature. But more than that, they provide individuals, especially younger ones, with a clear sense of self.

Telling athletes they need to retire from their sports for any reason can lead to sleepless nights, anxiety, and depression. These problems can then lead to cognitive concerns described as "fogginess" or short-term memory problems. Patients who are prone to headaches will have those too. If these symptoms aren't examined carefully and critically, they could easily be blamed on a recent concussion. The patient's fate becomes sealed when it is assumed that all of their symptoms are from head trauma, ignoring the potential contributions from being forced to retire.

This is not a rare situation. It comes up in our clinic multiple times every single week. Patients who have been told they can no longer play their sports suffer because of that determination, not because of any injury.

We will explore in the pages to follow the significant, sometimes life-altering negative effects of prematurely retiring from sports without a legitimate reason. At the same time, there can be very deep and harmful effects from getting your brain rattled too many times. My job, and the job of every concussion clinician, should be to understand both sides of this equation in order to do what's best for the patient. Whether an athlete can return to playing a sport after a concussion or should hang up his or her cleats is a complex medical decision that should not be made lightly.

The aim of this book is to have a serious, evidence-based discussion about the complicated relationships among sports, concussion, and the world we live in. Think of it as us sitting down for coffee and talking about this issue in a friendly and relaxed setting. My approach is based on my roles in life as a doctor, clinician, parent, and somebody who cares about athletes and sports. In no way is this book intended to replace the advice of your physician or neurologist; please be sure to continue consulting your physician and take her or his advice. It's my hope that after you read this book, perhaps even a couple of times, I will have helped you understand concussion a bit better, and you will be more informed when speaking with your doctor and have a better understanding of their recommendations. It is also my desire to expose the complexities of sports concussion science and medicine as well as the roles that the media and pop culture play in shaping ideas and attitudes about all things concussion. I hope that by the end, you will come to agree with me that your life is not over just because you—or someone you know—has had a concussion.

Jeff Kutcher, MD

ONE

SPORTS CONCUSSION MYTHS
AND FEARS

Spencer Helgren, in many ways, saw himself as the classic kid who dreamed of stardom on the football field.

He loved everything about the sport—the competition, the bonds with his teammates and coaches, the weight room commitment, and the buzz he felt playing for his school, Westwood High in the small Upper Peninsula town of Ishpeming, Michigan. Football was a big part of his teen identity, his way of connecting to friends and high school, and his form of expression. And Ishpeming was a typical American small town, where the Friday night high school football games were woven into the social fabric of the community.

Everything changed for Spencer during his junior year of high school. As a linebacker, he was often involved in plays with hard collisions and take-down finishes. During an early-season Friday game in 2010, Spencer was concussed. The collision was a hard, helmet-to-helmet smack that left Spencer a little dazed.

But Spencer popped up and stayed in the game, shaking off the impact, his ingrained football toughness taking over. A few series later, Spencer was driven to the ground while covering a punt. He felt strange, knew something was wrong but wasn't quite sure what, and burst into tears while lying on the ground. He was confused and scared.

We now know Spencer's story is not that unusual. Concussions happen every day, without fail, given the 35 million or so youth athletes across America who compete in popular sports such as football, soccer, volleyball, and ice hockey.

These scenes from youth sports should seem familiar:

Two high school football players violently slam into each other after an amazing catch, both going down in an awkward-looking heap. The crowd gasps in shock. After a few seconds, both players pop up, like Spencer did initially, and look ready to go.

A third-grade soccer player heads the ball, with her solid pass leading to the game's first goal. Her parents gleefully cheer her accomplishment but are unable to spot their daughter's wincing from the header.

A junior high wrestler pins his opponent to the mat but in the process bends his neck awkwardly while trying to gain more leverage. He falls over and screams. His parents see the injury and consider not letting him wrestle anymore.

Which athlete just incurred a concussion and will be properly assessed and treated? Which athlete, along with his or her caring parents and coaches, will not realize a brain trauma may have just occurred?

"I never wanted to come out of any football game," Spencer says. "I loved to play and prided myself on being a hard worker. So there was no question, even though I had never cried during a game before, that I wanted to keep going. I didn't have the thought to say, 'OK, I think I am really hurt, I might have a concussion, so I should stop playing football now.'

"I know I was in denial about all of it. I was not going to let anything stop me from playing. I even prided myself on trying to be the hardest-working and toughest player at Westwood. I liked that people looked up to me for that."

SEEING THE WHOLE PICTURE

Spencer tells an all-too-common tale. He wanted to be tough. He thought he needed to be tough, because he wanted to be a strong player. The tradition of his sport, combined with the peer-enforced ethic, is to be tough. It didn't cross his mind to come out of the game because he felt he needed to be a leader. This is a common mindset in all sports, of course. But in cases like this, is it really the whole story? Isn't it also possible that Spencer, in an impaired state from his brain injury, didn't know any better and couldn't make a logical decision about his health?

These are some of the issues I deal with every day as a sports neurologist. I see the full spectrum of athletes in my practice: children just beginning to learn their sports, high school and collegiate athletes in peak condition, elite Olympic and professional athletes, and retired athletes of all types now concerned that their lives of sport participation have doomed their brains to an impaired fate. I listen to moms and dads who only want what's best for their son or daughter. They weigh the benefits of playing sports against the mounting fears of sports-related brain trauma and its long-term implications.

This much is clear: Each of these important groups has been inundated with concussion awareness messaging. In the past decade or so, the average level of awareness and concern about sports concussion has grown tremendously. I am no longer seeing patients or families who are unaware of concussion. I am now counseling parents who come at these issues with a degree of education on the subject, mainly derived from stories on television, blogs, and other forms of media.

The raised awareness from the media is largely positive. Most people would agree, I imagine, that more attention, more concern, and increased resources focused on sports concussion all combine to produce a more thoughtful approach to the injury and improved safety. However, is this messaging actually improving the overall health of our athletes? Have we really increased the overall level of sports concussion *knowledge* for the average parent, coach, or athlete? Or have we simply turned a brilliantly blinding light on a complex issue without taking the time to present a thoughtfully composed and accurate message?

The public now thinks it knows concussion. But what type of sports collision leads to a concussion? Shouldn't it be obvious? People seem to think so. Just from watching a play either live or on television, many people assume they know the diagnosis. I receive emails almost weekly with attached video clips of a violent play or fall and a message from the sender assuming that I'm going to agree that an obvious concussion has happened. I carefully watch each clip—of a big football hit, a hockey fight, or a lacrosse player slammed from behind—and I try to put myself there on the sideline or behind the bench. I've been there enough to know this reality: Videos often tell only a part of the story. Unless you are there as a trained physician and evaluate the patient for yourself, you're only venturing a guess as to a diagnosis.

Often, these injury clips are sent with detailed and passionate comments on the dangers of athletics, and specifically contact-driven sports. I've been told more than once that sports such as boxing, mixed martial arts, and football should be banned to protect our athletes.

The phrase "How could they miss it?" is usually invoked in some form as well. The audience is now actively looking to spot concussions on the field of play. They assume the eye sees the concussion—and sometimes it does. But what we witness, either live or on video, does not necessarily line up with what is actually happening medically.

The idea that every big hit or violent fall will create a concussion is inaccurate. Even the "obvious" cases are sometimes misleading. The reality is, diagnosing a concussion is not as simple as watching a video clip or a report on ESPN. The camera only can give you only so much.

The confusion and concern surrounding sports concussion feed an increasingly energetic national conversation, one with a growing sensationalist narrative of doom and despair. You can't help but hear or read incorrect or simplistic assumptions, unwarranted conclusions, and myths repeated as fact.

Much of the attention comes from fears over the long-term health of our athletes, regardless of age. This is where things get still more complicated. Whatever the actual risks are to long-term brain health from playing sports, concussions themselves may not even be the biggest concern. They certainly aren't the only variable in play.

The heartfelt and tragic stories of athletes dealing with mental illness or who commit suicide drive the conversation to emotional places. From there, it's an easy leap to concluding that contact sports such as American football must be a dangerous endeavor, leading only to pain and even death. This relationship seems like fact only because anybody with a little knowledge—and sometimes a lot of agenda or a desire to gin up false debate—can get on television or radio or go on a Twitter rant to vent their thoughts to a large audience without challenge or fact-checking.

So why should you listen to—much less believe—somebody who's writing a book about concussions and athlete brain health? Good question!

My goal is to bring the issues behind this current discussion fully to life for you, with my sincere hope being that by the end of it, I will have provided enough wisdom and perspective to let you judge for yourself.

NOT A SIMPLE ISSUE

By now you've probably heard any number of experts trying to explain a concussion. On the one hand, the idea is simple: Your brain experiences enough force to cause you to feel bad. On the other hand, if only it *were* that simple. Not every hit to the head that causes a symptom means a concussion has occurred. At the same time, not every injury results from the brain's experiencing force will cause any symptoms. Sometimes it isn't clear for several hours that an injury has occurred.

Yet the current common expectation seems to be that a concussion should—even *must*—be diagnosed immediately after it occurs. And the new prevailing wisdom dictates that all athletes should be prevented from continuing to play after they have been diagnosed with a concussion. That would be a great idea, if it were at all attainable. Every day, I guarantee you, athletes and non-athletes alike continue with their normal courses of business after being injured.

Why do they do this? And how is it allowed to happen?

First, there is no way of demonstrating for sure with any medical test that a concussion has occurred, even though on some level we understand that somebody is either injured or not. Because not all brain injuries will produce symptoms, there will be times that injuries go undetected. Moreover, the signs and symptoms of concussion are variable, and not specific to concussion alone. There are dozens of potential alternative medical explanations for many of the symptom presentations of concussion. Non-clinicians will commonly declare that this seems impossible, saying, "Surely there must be a way to accurately diagnose a concussion." But diagnosing a concussion is not like being pregnant. I can't prove it on the spot by a simple blood test, an ultrasound, or having you pee on a stick.

Second, concussed people are, quite commonly, confused people. They often do not have intact thought processes. In other words, they are impaired. So when we ask a wide receiver who just got "rocked" while trying to make a catch over the middle if he is OK and he says, "Yeah, I'm good to go," we shouldn't necessarily believe it. He's not necessarily lying or hiding his symptoms to stay in the game. He may simply be unaware of the injury.

Putting these concepts together, I submit that while we always want to diagnose concussion quickly and accurately, it is far more important to focus on how we manage our patients in these situations. It doesn't really matter what the exact diagnosis is at any specific point in time. Rather, the important thing is that I treat you *as if* you are concussed—until it is clear that you're not.

Concussions produce nuanced neurological symptoms, presenting—and resolving—in individual ways. Concussion is not a one-size-fits-all, black-or-white, yes-or-no injury. We live in a world transformed by quick diagnostic answers, from a broken bone revealed on an X-ray to results from complex tests being run in mere hours. We rely on smartphones, computers, and Siri to give us answers mere seconds after we ask the questions. Not knowing something conclusively and immediately goes increasingly against what we have come to expect in other aspects of our lives.

Much of the public discussion of concussions doesn't help either. The terminology used to talk about concussions is often inaccurate. Causing further confusion, lingering, chronic issues after concussion are often not the direct results of the concussion at all.

GIVE IT TO ME STRAIGHT!

Simply put, a concussion is a type of a traumatic brain injury resulting from incidents involving direct—or indirect—blows to the head. Concussions can come from forces like a shove, leading to whiplash to the neck or back, or any other movement that jars the brain by making it move and stop quickly. Concussion is truly a universal injury: It can happen at any age, to males or females of any ethnicity, in any sport, at any time during a pickup game, organized practice, or competition. Wearing the newest equipment, buying the most expensive helmet, going for the latest gadget touted to monitor the brain, playing cautiously, working on excellent conditioning and technique, receiving the best training from great coaches, and having skilled medical staff on the sidelines may all help improve overall safety, but these things cannot prevent concussions from occurring. There is no physical sport that can be truthfully touted as "concussion free."

Concussion symptoms typically resolve in less than two weeks, but the concussion isn't necessarily over when the symptoms are. The injury may continue, producing symptoms only when the injured person resumes increased levels of physical and cognitive exertion. At the same time, not all of the symptoms a person experiences while concussed are necessarily due to the concussion itself. Factors such as sleep deprivation, depression, anxiety, and neck injury can all be concurrent causes of symptoms after a concussion.

For these reasons, concussed athletes need to be under the care of knowledgeable and experienced medical professionals, who can implement and properly monitor a thoughtful approach to healing and a safe return to play.

DRAWING SOME IMPORTANT DISTINCTIONS

The term *concussion* is most commonly used throughout our society to cover any negative brain health effect that might occur as a result of being hit. The player who misses one week with a concussion, the patient who experienced three months of headaches and foggy thinking, and the former star player now concerned about his memory are all thought to have "concussion problems." This is not accurate.

"Concussion" should be used only to specifically describe the injury that is a direct result of the insulting force or the clinical effect of that injury. In the overwhelming majority (over 80%) of cases, the clinical effect of a concussion is over in two to three weeks. To be clear, concussions rarely last longer than two to three weeks, but they can, especially if there is a complication, such as another hit or continued strenuous physical or cognitive exertion.

Sometimes, however, symptoms continue beyond the typical two or three weeks. In these cases, symptoms may represent the effects of a longer-than-usual concussion, or they may not actually be from the concussion itself but rather may result from a complex interaction of multiple factors. This second situation is best described as *post-concussion syndrome*, and while treating it can be difficult, it is absolutely treatable. Therefore the patient who's been experiencing symptoms for several months is most likely no longer concussed but rather has post-concussion syndrome. This distinction is extremely important, as the medical management of these two entities is very different.

A final distinction to keep in mind has to do with the increasingly common stories of former athletes, especially those who participated in contact sports, having problems with their thinking, mood, and memory later in life. Media reports tell stories of star athletes who are dealing with a concussion as a long-term medical issue. The truth is, they are no longer concussed. They may have a serious neurological condition as a result of playing sports, but it is not concussion. Their history of diagnosed concussions—how many they had and when—may not even be as important as how often they were hit.

So while it is convenient that we have one term to describe all of the things that make up the spectrum of traumatically induced brain health problems (after all, it's in the title of this book), we need to be very careful to not mix things up too much. That's how the messages provided by the media and others can become misleading and even harmful. These issues require a much more critical thought process than you typically hear in 10-second sound bites.

The majority of this book, especially the next few chapters, focuses on concussion itself. Post-concussion syndrome and the long-term effects of playing sports will also be addressed, of course.

POP CULTURE AND MEDICAL MEMES

What concussions are—and more importantly, what they are not—is becoming more confused and muddled in the at-large conversation about sports, concussions, and athletes. The murkiness in facts and messaging leaves parents, coaches, and athletes in an uncomfortable limbo. They are being influenced by information that is not medically sound and are now often choosing to preemptively limit an athlete's participation in sports out of a fear of concussions that is based on question-able assumptions.

Parental peer pressure is spreading. "Youth football is too dangerous" and "Three concussions and you're done" are common memes. More and more frequently I even hear warn-ings like "Don't let your child play soccer, because they will get a concussion and become neurologically compromised for life."

This tangible mounting fear of concussion is changing the landscape of youth sports. There has been a dramatic societal shift in the 2000s, from an overall lack of awareness about concussions in athletes at the start of the new century to a near-stigmatizing panic about the injury a decade later. Concussions and related brain health issues are now viewed as certain out-comes from athletic participation at any level.

It's important to understand both what we know about concussions and what remains medically and scientifically un-known. Concussions themselves are not life-threatening, and the vast majority of them do not automatically put an end to future athletic participation. Yet a growing number of parents are having their children avoid participating in contact sports such as football or ice hockey to "protect" them from concus-sion. If the right measures are in place, that drastic step is un-necessary.

In fact, I'd argue, being overprotective for no reason can be detrimental in other ways. Being involved in sports is a normal, positive activity for youth and adults, promoting good health, emotional and mental release, and personal growth through human interaction. Whether on a Little League diamond or the local YMCA basketball court, being athletic adds to the quality of childhood experiences and forms a critical part of living a healthy life.

Learning the satisfaction and rewards of doing your best, working with your teammates, learning new skills, and, yes, winning a game or a trophy are powerful childhood experiences. We also recall the failures, those painful moments when we let in a big goal or missed a tackle in a close game. Embracing the joys and coping with the defeats are important childhood touchstones, and although we need to promote safety above all, I hope they are not bypassed because of irrational fears of injury.

All of these factors, and more, should go into the complex equation of when to go back to a sport after a concussion (or any other serious injury) and when to retire.

MORE THAN JUST A CONTACT SPORT PROBLEM

We've all seen the bone-crunching plays that lead to concussions in contact sports like football and ice hockey.

But what about an elbow to the side of the head while rebounding in a basketball game? Or the searing volleyball spike that ricochets off a teammate's hand into the middle blocker's face? The snowboarder who tries a new trick off a rail but lands awkwardly and slaps her head back on the packed snow? We need to reconsider seemingly more innocent things as well, such as the cheerleader who accidentally falls after a tumbling pass or the diver who misaligns his head and misses a clean entry into the water.

They all could also be concussed, even if we didn't "see" it.

Contrary to what was once a popular assumption, most concussions occur without a loss of consciousness. Too many in the public still cling to the outdated notion that the biggest diagnostic clues to concussion are being "knocked out" or being "out cold." More commonly, concussions produce only momentary disorientation or a brief interruption in memory. Momentary disorientation, often described by the old cliché of "getting your bell rung," can signal that some form of neurological impairment may have occurred—even if consciousness was not lost.

It used to be a badge of athletic pride to say you shook off being hurt or in pain and kept playing. Parents and coaches have encouraged players, sometimes in adamant ways, to "shake it off" and keep going after being slammed to the turf. We celebrate athletes who went on to do "heroic" things after they were knocked out, dazed, or dizzy to the point of being nauseated. For them, leaving the game or admitting they were hurt was not an option. They prioritized their teammates, winning, their careers, or even their own egos as athletes above their health.

But hearing the arena or field's disc jockey play Taylor Swift's "Shake It Off" after somebody gets hurt does not send the most apt message for injury awareness. The advancement of medical science tells us that playing through dizziness, nausea, disorientation, or other symptoms yields no neurological dividends for the athlete's long-term health. Those signs of impairment indicate that something serious has occurred and needs to be professionally evaluated. We've also learned that concussions are not reserved for professional athletes or competitors for Olympic gold medals.

CONCUSSIONS THROUGH
THE YEARS

Concussions have been a described medical issue since at least the days of the ancient Greeks, whose famous medical writings described impaired speech, sight, and mental function as consequences of brain injury. The first acknowledged medical professional to write extensively about concussion as a medical issue was Muhammad ibn Zakariya al-Razi, a Persian doctor of the mid-9th to mid-10th century A.D. who described the injury as a serious form of brain trauma. The word *concussion* itself, from Latin roots meaning "violent shaking," entered the medical literature by the mid-17th century.[1]

The connection between sports and head trauma came into sharper focus in more recent times. In the strange way that history seems to frequently repeat itself, we can go back to the early 1900s for an earlier wave of concern about football, then under fire for being too dangerous. National discussion centered on the violence of the game, which was then more about pushing and shoving, often in big piles of players, to gain field position and protect the ball. Players did not wear helmets or the array of gladiator-like protective equipment donned by today's players at all levels.

Eight players died, and over 100 were injured, playing football in 1905 alone. The October 15, 1905, edition of the *Washington Post* reported 45 players died from head trauma, internal trauma, or spinal injuries from 1900 to 1905.[2] Charles Eliot, then president of Harvard University, described football as "more brutalizing than prizefighting, cockfighting or bullfighting" and was considering ending his school's program.[3] Columbia, Duke, and Northwestern had already decided to end their football programs over concerns about the safety of their student–athletes.

President Theodore Roosevelt was a big football fan and was reported to be quite alarmed at the growing rate of grave, life-threatening injuries. He also saw that an anti-football movement was on the rise because of those injuries. He asked the presidents of Yale, Princeton, and Harvard (where his own son, Theodore Jr., was a freshman football player) to meet at the White House to consider reforms.[4] A *New-York Tribune* article discussed Roosevelt's desire to find a compromise to save football by a "lessening of brutality" in the game.[5]

(Truth be told, Roosevelt, who never played college football, loved the physicality of the game. He wasn't looking to change football too much and was quoted as saying at a Harvard Club banquet in the 1890s, "What matters a few broken bones to the glories of intercollegiate sport?"[6])

What came out of that meeting was the momentum to create the Intercollegiate Athletic Association of the United States, the forerunner to today's NCAA, and to mandate greater safety measures, such as wearing helmets, to preserve football.

Boxing moved into the spotlight next, thanks to its increasing popularity as a sport whose practitioners delivered—and received—repeated blows to the head. Boxers were studied and became the first recognized athlete group to be assessed as having a new, sports-related neurodegenerative disease, dementia pugilistica. This disorder was introduced into the medical literature in 1928 by Dr. Harrison Stanford Martland, who described it using the common term "punch drunk."[7] Boxers with dementia pugilistica looked and acted drunk, even though they were technically sober, because of the brain trauma from boxing.

The concept of a relationship among sports, head trauma, and possibly lasting neurological consequences started to become clearer.

Still, even with ongoing research, the worlds of medicine and sports didn't know what to advocate as best practices for athlete health. A 1952 study in the *New England Journal of Medicine* advocated for athletes to retire after a third concussion.[8] The practice of grading concussions by degree of severity (which is no longer used) started in 1986. In 1990 the

Colorado Medical Society released the first set of working guidelines for sports concussion management, which spread throughout collegiate and high school sports medicine.[9] The Colorado guidelines helped establish the concept of standardizing how long to sit players out following a concussion, providing a range of one week to one year depending on the concussion's severity (then called its grade). The guidelines and their dissemination didn't have the same impact as the creation of the NCAA's forerunner and later the NCAA, but they were a step forward in taking concussions more seriously on a wider scale.

This development was only the beginning of increased concussion awareness and attempts to find "protocols" to help physicians manage concussion. The sports medicine world has come a long way in the past 10 years, and our understanding of the best practices for managing these injuries continues to evolve.

CONCUSSIONS MOVE INTO THE MAINSTREAM

Thanks to research stemming from the concern over boxing and football brain trauma nine decades ago, medicine has become more aware of the potential for serious brain impairments from playing sports. But the carryover of strong concussion awareness and medically established knowledge about concussion to other sports, especially those played by children, has been slower and a bit more convoluted.

Globally, the fields of neurological science and medicine, and their army of researchers, have all been chasing the same big idea: how to unlock the secrets of the brain. We're all running on parallel tracks, often weaving together, to understand this most complex of organs. So many medical issues relating to concussion in particular still need to be unpacked with good evidence. Why do similar blows to the head, like headers in soccer, affect one player quite adversely and leave another unscathed? Why do some people seem to be immune to impacts while others develop symptoms from even a minor bump?

The pendulum of public awareness has swung dramatically in the last decade, from concussions not regarded as a significant problem to them now causing great fear among many people. Unfortunately, these two positions are equally flawed. It's irresponsible to remain uninformed about concussions, and it's wrong to minimize their impact on our athletes. Concussions must be assessed, treated, and managed correctly. However, they usually do not need to be the automatic end of an athlete's career nor a prevailing reason to preemptively avoid sports.

The past 20 years of neurological research and clinical experience have taught us that concussions from athletic pursuits at any age or level must be taken seriously. According to a 2010 study by the Centers for Disease Control and Prevention, [10] nearly 2.7 million youth athletes under the age of 19 were treated in emergency rooms for sports-related injuries from 2001 to 2009. Concussions and traumatic brain injuries accounted for 6.5 percent, or 173,285, of those injuries. When the data is broken down, it shows that the rate of ER visits went up 62 percent over that nine-year span, from 153,375 in 2001 to 248,418 in 2009.

Such an increase is hard to ignore, but why did it happen? Did our sports, especially our contact sports, change that much in just eight years? Sure, they may have changed a little during that time. Athletes may be playing more aggressively, and thanks to training techniques making them stronger and faster, impact forces may be more significant too. Some players are also looking to make a name for themselves as tough or intimidating, developing that reputation through those jaw-dropping "big hits" that make ESPN's famous "SportsCenter" highlight lists or go viral on YouTube.

But the common thinking, with which I certainly agree, is that most of this increase in concussions reflects a different approach to the injury, including increased general awareness and a lower threshold of when to suspect it. There is a sense that the concussion rates that have been reported since roughly 2009 likely reflect a more accurate estimation of the true number of injuries than do past figures.

On the other hand, I must caution that because diagnosing concussion is not always black or white, the dramatic shift in public awareness has likely increased the number of "false positive" diagnoses—those situations where concussion is diagnosed as the cause of a patient's symptoms when in fact they have another origin.

From a public health perspective, I would argue that it is good to have some false positives, to ensure that we're capturing as many of the actual concussions as possible. We must also realize, however, that a false positive diagnosis may also cause harm to the individual who receives it. We need to strive to be as good as we can about getting diagnosis right.

CHANGING, DYNAMIC SYMPTOMS

The play on the football field, soccer pitch, or gymnastics mat that results in a concussion starts a series of physiological changes in the brain. These changes cause dysfunction of the brain's cells, the neurons, which in turn leads to the signs and symptoms of concussion. The type of signs and degree of symptoms are varied and unique to each injury. When function is disturbed in this way, symptoms can evolve and shift as the brain tries to deal with the injury.

Sometimes the symptoms go away within moments, disappearing as abruptly as they began. Other times, symptoms such as headache or nausea develop over minutes or hours. What is important at these early stages is that a trained and experienced medical professional, such as a certified athletic trainer, primary care sports medicine physician, or a sports neurologist like myself, must be able to comprehensively assess the athlete. Essential components of safeguarding athlete health include understanding these complex medical scenarios, possessing the skills to assess potential injuries, understanding when there is medical cause to remove an athlete from play, and having good, informed judgment about when to pursue further avenues of medical care.

Unfortunately, not every high school and not many youth sports programs have a physician at games, let alone practices. Even more concerning, as of 2012, less than half of U.S. high schools had access to a full- or part-time athletic trainer.[11] As a result, a coach or parent is often the first line of evaluation for a possible concussion.

Knowing what is happening to the athlete, how to correctly assess potential injuries, having the understanding of when to medically remove them from play, and perhaps pursuing further avenues of medical care, are all essential components to safeguarding athlete health.

Remember Spencer, the high school football player we met earlier? On that autumn Friday night when he collided with a member of the opposing team, he was evaluated after the game by his school's athletic trainer and cleared to resume working out and practicing. The next morning he showed up as usual for his team's Saturday morning weight lifting session. He loved the bonding time with his teammates, and the weightlifting workout was also a fun macho competition for him and his friends. Spencer felt fine when he started his first reps, but he soon became dizzy. He felt like he wanted to throw up when he tried to clear heavier weights over his head. Spencer seemed to be struggling, to the degree that his coach noticed. They addressed his shaky condition and decided he should sit out the rest of the weightlifting session.

Spencer recovered from his wave of nausea and grew steadier and stronger during the next week. He played in his team's game that Friday. Things took a scary turn during the game, leaving Spencer feeling like he was living in a rerun. He went to make a tackle and experienced his second helmet-to-helmet collision in a week. This time, he quickly realized he was probably dealing with another concussion.

"I have a great memory, I typically know everything that has happened around me in a game, and I knew now that all the signs were pointing to me having a concussion," Spencer says. "But I couldn't be in denial anymore. I knew something was wrong."

He had suffered three separate blows to his head in the span of a week, with each making his concussion worse. Now his brain was showing the cumulative effects. Spencer became sensitive to light and sound and plunged into a nonstop, 24-hour cycle of painful headaches that lasted for six months. He admits he felt depressed and scared, worried that something was seriously wrong—and that he would never be well or be able to return to football.

His family and friends also openly worried about him, begging him to give up any thoughts of playing football in his senior year. They thought football was too dangerous and he should spend his last year of high school concentrating on his studies and other activities.

PLAYING THROUGH PAIN?

We now know that playing with a concussion, either moments after it happens or days later, while the brain is still healing, can lead to more serious issues and longer injuries. Repeated blows to the head can result in serious brain trauma, cognitive and psychological issues, and even permanent impairment.

While the public has become more receptive to discussing concussions as an issue in sports, the facts of the discussion can become garbled. We have all been exposed to heartbreaking tales of athletes, from retired NFL stars Dave Duerson and Junior Seau to Ohio State reserve football player Kosta Karageorge, who were assumed to have had concussions and then committed suicide because of depression. Stories of living famous athletes claiming to have been diagnosed with chronic traumatic encephalopathy (CTE), which can lead to memory loss, confusion, and depression, splash across newspaper sports section headlines and take top billing on TV shows. Some players who die, some of them by suicide, are also declared with great fanfare to have gotten CTE from concussions. Despite this compelling narrative, the reality is that concussions and long-term effects like CTE are completely different processes that may not even be closely related.

These sensationalistic stories certainly tug at the heart-strings, especially when they are about a favorite player. But there is a big problem: Medically, we are not even close to understanding all the connections that might exist among sports, concussions, depression, suicide, and CTE.

Linking concussions with suicides is tenuous and, in a greater sense, also quite irresponsible. The issue is much more complex than that. Issues like depression, substance abuse, chronic pain, and even sleep apnea may underlie many athletes' suicides, just as they do those of non-athletes.

Having an improved awareness and respect for concussions in athletes as a serious medical issue is a tremendous step forward. This improved awareness is a positive in the growth of the medical community and the education of the public at large. But the outgrowth of kids being held out of sports because of fears over concussion, as seen by the continued downturn in participation in Pop Warner football, is a sad development for everybody.

Staying away from sports because of fear of concussions based on bad or incomplete knowledge is not a decision I can support as a neurologist. Sports can and should be part of the life of every child who wants to be an athlete. Getting a concussion does not have to be a sign of impending doom. Most of my patients recover fully and move on with their lives, resuming sports at their own levels.

That's what lies behind the goal of this book: Be real about concussions and athletics. Talk about the risks, about how to deal with injury, and about how, hopefully, to get back into play.

But what about Spencer? He overcame his concussions and returned to his everyday life. He found his way to our clinic, where a treatment plan and a few months of recovery brought him back to better brain function and to the sport he loves. He played football his final year of high school, did not get hurt, and received first-team all-league honors in 2011. The fears of his friends and family were allayed, and Spencer says he was able to achieve his own peace of mind through being able to play football with his friends his senior year.

Spencer currently attends college, has a normal, healthy life, and hopes to become a chiropractor. He freely speaks out about concussions in sports, wanting others to understand the need to take the issue seriously. He stays active through working out and recreational sports, and he says he doesn't fear for his future because he has had concussions.

"It was super scary to go through that, and at the time, I thought I would never be right," Spencer says. "But I am fine. I am not scared about what happened to me, because it was an injury, I got treatment, I healed, and my life goes on.

"People need to understand that getting a concussion, or even a few like me, doesn't mean the end of your life. You just need to take it seriously and get the right help to get well. I know I am happy that I was able to come back and not give in to being afraid of playing football and getting hurt."

REFERENCES

1. McCrory PR, Berkovic, SF. Concussion: The history of clinical and pathophysiological concepts and misconceptions. *Neurology* 2001;57(12):2283–2289.
2. Zezima K. How Teddy Roosevelt helped save football. *Washington Post.* May 29, 2014. http://www.washingtonpost.com/blogs/the-fix/wp/2014/05/29/teddy-roosevelt-helped-save-football-with-a-white-house-meeting-in-1905.
3. Klein C. How Teddy Roosevelt saved football. http://www.history.com/news/how-teddy-roosevelt-saved-football. September 6, 2012.
4. Hears football men; coaches in conference with President Roosevelt. Would put end to brutality. *Washington Post.* October 10, 1905. https://www.documentcloud.org/documents/1175005-144576144-1.html.
5. *New-York Tribune.* December 13, 1905. *Chronicling America: Historic American Newspapers.* Library of Congress.
6. Beschloss M. T.R.'s son inspired him to help rescue football. *New York Times.* August 1, 2014. http://www.nytimes.com/2014/08/02/upshot/trs-son-inspired-him-to-help-rescue-football.html.
7. Martland HS. Punch drunk. *Journal of the American Medical Association* 1928;91(15):1103–1107.
8. Thorndike A. Serious recurrent injuries of athletes; contraindications to further competitive participation. *New England Journal of Medicine* 1952;247(15):554–556.
9. Colorado Medical Society School and Sports Medicine Committee.

Guidelines for the management of concussion in sports. *Colorado Medicine* 1990;87:4.

10. Faul M, Xu L, Wald MM, Coronado VG. *Traumatic Brain Injury in the United States: Emergency Department Visits, Hospitalizations and Deaths 2002–2006.* Atlanta, GA: National Center for Injury Prevention and Control, Centers for Disease Control and Prevention, US Dept. of Health and Human Services; 2010.

11. National Athletic Trainers' Association. www.nata.org. 2013.

Two

Athletes, Concussions, and the Playing Field

Conduct a simple experiment with your friends and family: Ask them what sports they think carry the highest rates of concussion for children.

I bet the answers will come quickly.

> Football. Soccer. Maybe somebody will throw ice hockey or boxing.
> Follow up with another question: *Who* do they think is getting the concussions?
> Boys? Girls? Athletes of both genders equally?
> Preschoolers? Middle schoolers? Only the high school stars looking to play varsity in college or go pro?

The answers are most likely to fall along similar lines, with teen boys mentioned as at highest risk. Then girls will be brought up, occasionally, as getting concussions too.

And in two short questions, you will have uncovered the main issues that need to be addressed in our evolving journey of improving concussion awareness and the medical treatment of youth athletes.

There's no question that concussions occur in football and soccer. And when we think about football, it is obviously primarily a male sport. The narrative of NFL and college football being the main source of concussions is everywhere and carries a lot of influence over how the public perceives the issue.

But what about the globally popular sports of soccer and ice hockey? Or lacrosse? Diving? Wrestling? Cheerleading? Basketball? Mixed martial arts? Snowboarding? Gymnastics? Volleyball? Softball?

I think you get my point. The lines are not nearly as neat as we'd like them to be, and there is no axiom saying playing sport X guarantees that a concussion will—or will not—occur. I wish I could tell you a sport where concussions will never, ever happen. Avoiding all risk is impossible, and sports, like life in general, are a risk-versus-reward proposition.

We shouldn't assume, for example, that boys who don't try out for the high school football team but play soccer instead will never be concussed. Or that steering girls away from headers in soccer or spikes in volleyball will guarantee that those sports will be concussion free. The assumptions break down further in artistic sports such as cheerleading, which some people assume to be quite safe because there is no tackling, no moving bats or sticks, and no jarring play. But the act of stunting, where a cheerleader (called a flyer) is tossed upwards of a story into the air to perform an acrobatic move and then caught by her teammates (the base), can lead to concussions for all involved if not executed cleanly and with skill.

FEAR OF CONCUSSION AFFECTS
SPORTS PARTICIPATION

Parents, who often volunteer as youth coaches for their children's sports teams, have heard of concussion but are unable to accurately pin down what the injury is or who can get hurt. Still, they are starting to make their own conclusions about sports participation based on their perceptions of concussion risk. An Associated Press/GfK poll conducted during July 2014 revealed that out of 1,000 parents of youth athletes, 44 percent were "not comfortable" with their children playing football because of the possibility of concussions. Forty-five percent were not comfortable with their children taking part in wrestling, and 44 percent had concerns about ice hockey.[1]

In a 2013 HBO Real Sports/Marist University survey, 56 percent of the American adults queried said the possibility of neurological injury from playing football would be one of the deciding factors in determining if their child could participate. Sixteen percent said the risk of neurological injury from football would the primary factor in deciding whether or not their child could participate.[2]

It's encouraging that other sports, such as baseball/softball, soccer, swimming, track and field, and basketball, do not set off such alarm among surveyed parents. One study, conducted in September 2014 by espnW (ESPN's women's sports arm) and the Aspen Institute's Sports and Society Program,[3] addressed its questions to parents of children under 18. Eighty percent let their kids play some form of sport.

Still, injuries are a big parental concern, as 87 percent of the parents in that survey said they were worried about their children being injured playing sports. As Figure 2.1 shows, concussion was the kind of injury that well over half of mothers were most concerned about, while more than 40 percent of fathers cited concussion as their biggest injury fear.

So the majority of parents are not keeping their children out of sports because of concussion risk. Even so, overall youth participation in team sports is shrinking. In the United States, according to a January 2014 article in the *Wall Street Journal*,[4]

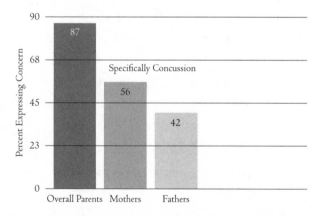

Figure 2.1 In a 2014 survey, 87 percent of parents of children under 18 were concerned that their children could be injured while playing sports. Among possible injuries, concussion was of the most concern to 56 percent of mothers and 42 percent of fathers. (Data from espnW/Aspen Institute Sport and Society Program, "Project Play Survey of Parents on Youth Sports Issues," September 2014.)

the top four youth sports—baseball, basketball, football, and soccer—all saw significant drops in participation by kids ages 6–17 from 2008 to 2012. As Figure 2.2 shows, basketball dropped the most, by over 8 percent, followed in order by baseball, soccer, and football.

Not all of the decreases in participation can be attributed to concussion concerns. Today's kids are more and more into video and interactive gaming as a recreational activity. And curiously, two of the more potentially concussion-prone sports, ice hockey and lacrosse, saw significant gains in youth participation. Ice hockey jumped by more than 60 percent from 2008

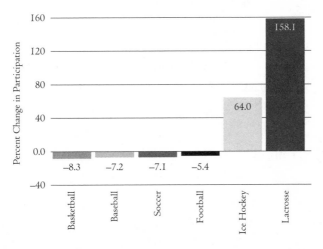

Figure 2.2 From 2008 to 2012, participation in baseball, basketball, football, and soccer by children ages 6–17 decreased significantly. At the same time, the historically less popular sports of ice hockey and, especially, lacrosse saw strong percentage increases. (Data from R. Wallerson, "Youth participation weakens in basketball, football, baseball, soccer," *Wall Street Journal*, January 1, 2014.)

to 2012, while lacrosse was up by a staggering 158 percent. Lacrosse's especially quick growth among youth is reflected in the rise from only 5,000 registered participants in 2001 to 403,770 in 2013, according to statistics gathered by US Lacrosse.[5]

All of these numbers on participation, of course, reflect multiple factors, including a sport's popularity, affordability, and accessibility. Still, it does seem that fear of concussions is making a significant contribution.

SPORTS = CONCUSSION RISK

Overall, 7.8 million teens participate in all forms of high school sports. There are a lot of kids involved in organized team sport activities outside of school as well as the traditionally non-school-based sports such as gymnastics, figure skating, and skateboarding. According to USA Football, nearly 1.1 million students play high school football, and a total of 3 million children are involved in all levels of youth football.[6] In 2012, more than 3 million children played on teams organized by US Youth Soccer. Even with the drop in soccer participation mentioned above, that's a dramatic change from when statistics were first compiled for soccer in 1974, when only 104,000 kids played.[7]

Which of these activities lead to the most concussions? In studies published in 2011 and 2012 in the *American Journal of Sports Medicine*, a few sports led the way in concussion rates among high school athletes. Football was number one, followed by boys' ice hockey, boys' and girls' soccer, boys' and girls' lacrosse, boys' wrestling, boys' and girls' basketball, girls' softball, and cheerleading.[8,9] (Sports in which both boys and girls participate, such as soccer and basketball, were combined for list-making brevity.) About 30 percent of the participants reported having had two or more concussions during the school year covered by one of these surveys.[10] The athletes had varied participation levels, from starters to the kids at the end of the bench who practiced more than they ever played in games.

A growing amount of studies are starting to reveal how youth athletes are getting concussed in different sports. A 2007 study showed that tackling or being tackled in football accounted for 67.6 percent of concussions in high school athletes.[11] A study published in 2009 in the *Journal of Athletic Training* tracked falls and injuries among 412 cheerleaders in the United States during the 2006–07 school year. Stunting or forming a pyramid accounted for 70 of the 79 fall-related injuries recorded. Six percent of the injuries were concussions.[12]

So you can see that by considering only the obvious sports, you get only part of the story and miss the larger picture of who is at risk. The complete story is much more nuanced and inclusive: Concussions can happen at any time, in any sport, in numerous ways. They can happen without contact, and they can happen after a nasty takedown. Concussions, and the ways they happen in athletics, can be as individual as the athletes themselves. Many factors come into play: How strong is the athlete's neck against whiplash-like blows? Is there a family history of migraine headaches or sleep problems? Does the athlete have preexisting sensitivities to light, sound, or other sensory issues? Is the sport itself inherently risky, like snowboarding or X Games–style competitions, leading competitors to push the edges of safety for higher scores or faster times?

Now think about factors affecting the child athlete. Coaching, technique, coordination, level of aggression, the type of refereeing (lax enforcement or strictly by the book), and developmental stage all can contribute to determining who is at higher risk of becoming concussed. A lot of dynamic factors are swirling around, and few are truly controllable.

Pete Vaz, a longtime high school basketball coach in California, says he wonders what he should be looking for to protect his athletes from concussions. He has experienced the evolution from parents' not knowing anything about concussion to concerned moms and dads now asking him frequent questions about their child's health after a collision.

"I really have seen parents change in the last five, six years, because I hear the questions they ask me or the trainers," says Vaz. "I think it is a really good development. I am happy that we're all looking out for the players, because that's what we're supposed to do. But it is something that is also challenging, because I don't feel like I have all the answers I need to have sometimes."

MORE CONCUSSIONS, OR MORE
CONCUSSION AWARENESS?

Dr. Christopher Giza, a world-renowned neurologist at the University of California, Los Angeles, who specializes in developmental traumatic brain injury, says understanding how children are affected by concussion is a growing field of scientific study and knowledge. Dr. Giza frequently lectures on concussion in children, emphasizing that concussed children need to be seen as their own class of patient—not as little adults with concussions. The age of the concussed child needs to be a strong consideration in how quickly that child can return to play, according to Dr. Giza: Younger children may need more time to recover from a concussion than teens.

"I think the awareness is increasing every day that children can be concussed from playing sports, and that is a big change from, say, 10 years ago, when people thought they didn't play sports at a physical enough level to get a brain injury," Dr. Giza says. "But there is still a lot of confusion on who is getting concussed, and I think the parents are now becoming reactive and fearful of certain sports like football. It's never been so easy that we could point the finger at one thing, and say, this is it—change this, and we eliminate concussions. I would love to make it like that, but that's not the world we live in."

Dr. Giza also brings up a good point about statistics from the 2010 Centers for Disease Control report showing ER visits

for sports- and recreation-related childhood concussions jumping by nearly 60 percent from 2002 to 2006.[13]

"Are our children getting more concussions from sports?
Or are we just getting stronger awareness and better abilities
to correctly diagnose children who are concussed from sports
injuries?" Dr. Giza asks. "I am leaning toward us getting better
in calling the concussions for what they are. We have increased
awareness, with parents, athletic trainers, doctors, and medical
personnel all looking for concussions.

"People are learning to ask the right questions and take
head injury seriously, which is a critical improvement. That's
one of the most positive changes I see, so yes, it probably leads
to the numbers going up among the concussed."

At the same time, this increased awareness has led to more
things being called concussion that actually aren't. These false
positives are a natural product of increasing awareness and
concern.

What we should take away from all of this is that concussions do occur more often than we thought 10 years ago,
but because concussions continue to be difficult to diagnose
with absolute certainty and there is no objective test for the
injury, there remains a lot of ambiguity and a lot of un-
knowns.

"We need to be thoughtful about everything when it comes
to properly assessing children with concussions," Dr. Giza
says. "Being overprotective or overreactive, without the proper
evidence or cause, about concussion isn't the way we should be

going. We need to be safe, smart, and prepared to help children be involved in sports and have fun. That's always my goal, as both a physician and a parent."

THE QUESTION OF CTE

Another concern for parents and coaches with respect to concussions and sports centers around the risks of depression and CTE (chronic traumatic encephalopathy). Every day, news stories appear connecting concussion to depression and CTE, a progressive and incurable brain disease, in athletes. The media throw the acronym CTE around with only brief discussion, and little explanation, whenever autopsies of the brains of former star athletes are said to reveal it.

It's true that medicine knows that multiple blows to the head may lead to CTE. But this knowledge comes from quantitative research on individuals who have died. Though CTE is a permanent condition that develops over a lifetime, it cannot yet be accurately diagnosed in the living. Only upon death can the brain be dissected and examined closely to find evidence of the disease.

So the serious discussion about CTE becomes confused when athletes such as former NFL star quarterback Bernie Kosar and Hall of Fame running back Tony Dorsett[14] publicly state that they have been diagnosed with CTE or CTE-like symptoms. Any diagnosis of CTE is at best a guess, and at worst untrue speculation, until a person dies and his or her brain is examined.

Parents of youth athletes, and sometimes the athletes themselves, express fears that getting concussed means getting CTE, Alzheimer's disease, other kinds of dementia, or another serious progressive neurological disease. The vast majority of individuals who get concussions, upwards of 90 percent, recover fully, without further issues. It is the minority who transition into post-concussive syndromes, and an even rarer group whose injuries progress into the most serious neurological conditions.

In other words, if you do get a concussion, the odds are very much in your favor that you will recover fully. Obviously, being properly assessed and treated goes a long way in leveraging your odds for an optimal recovery.

Being afraid of the unknown and, at this point, unproven doesn't outweigh the good of participating in athletics in any form and at any level. The values learned, the joy in acquiring new skills, the fun of play, and the relationships and self-confidence built from youth sports should far outweigh fears of concussion.

REFERENCES

1. http://ap-gfkpoll.com/main/wp-content/uploads/2014/08/AP-GfK-July-2014-Poll-Topline-FINAL_Kids-sports.pdf.
2. Marist Poll. 10/23: Youth football takes hard hit…. One-third of Americans less likely to allow son to play football because of

head injury risk. October 22, 2013. http://maristpoll.marist.edu/ 1023-youth-football-takes-hard-hit-one-third-of-americans-less-likely-to-allow-son-to-play-football-because-of-head-injury-risk/.

3. espnW/Aspen Institute Sport and Society Program. Project Play survey of parents on youth sports issues. September 2014. http:// aspenprojectplay.org/sites/default/files/espnw-Aspen Institute Project Play Survey of Parents on youth sports issues.pdf.

4. Wallerson R. Youth participation weakens in basketball, football, baseball, soccer. *Wall Street Journal.* January 1, 2014. http://www.wsj. com/articles/SB10001424052702303519404579350892629229 918.

5. US Lacrosse. 2013 Participation survey. http://www.usla-crosse.org/Portals/1/documents/pdf/about-the-sport/2013-participation-survey.pdf.

6. Folio J. NFHS study: High school football participation numbers grew in 2013. August 22, 2014. http://usafootball.com/blogs/ americas-game/post/9257/nfhs-study:-high-school-football-participation-numbers-grew-in-2013.

7. US Youth Soccer. Key statistics. http://www.usyouthsoccer.org/ media_kit/keystatistics/

8. Meehan WP, d'Hemecourt P, Collins C, Comstock RD. Assessment and management of sport-related concussions in United States high schools. *American Journal of Sports Medicine* 2011;39(11):2304–2310.

9. Marar M, McIlvain NM, Fields SK, Comstock RD. Epidemiology of concussions among United States high school athletes in 20 sports. *American Journal of Sports Medicine* 2012;40(4):747–755.

10. Meehan WP, d'Hemecourt P, Collins C, Comstock RD. Assessment and management of sport-related concussions in United States high schools. *American Journal of Sports Medicine* 2011;39(11):2304–2310.

11. Gessel LM, Fields SK, Collins CL, Dick RW, Comstock RD. Concussions among United States high school and collegiate athletes. *Journal of Athletic Training* 2007;42(4):495–503.

12. Shields BJ, Smith GA. Epidemiology of cheerleading-related falls in the United States. *Journal of Athletic Training* 2009;44(6):578–85. doi:10.4085/1062-6050-44.6.578.

13. Faul M, Xu L, Wald MM, Coronado VG. *Traumatic Brain Injury in the United States: Emergency Department Visits, Hospitalizations and Deaths 2002–2006.* Atlanta, GA: National Center for Injury Prevention and Control, Centers for Disease Control and Prevention, US Dept. of Health and Human Services; 2010.

14. Weinbaum W, Delsohn S. Dorsett, others show signs of CTE. April 5, 2014. http://espn.go.com/espn/otl/story/_/id/9931754/former-nfl-stars-tony-dorsett-leonard-marshall-joe-delameilleure-show-indicators-cte-resulting-football-concussions.

THREE

YOU THINK YOU MIGHT HAVE A CONCUSSION—HOW DO YOU KNOW?

Things would be a lot easier if we had a quick, easy, and reliable test for concussion. Coaches, parents, and especially our patients would love to receive a red light/green light, yes-or-no, quick, and definitive diagnosis from the medical professionals evaluating them on the sidelines.

We are not there yet, medically or scientifically. Not even close. That was true the very first time I was asked to cover a college football game as a physician, over 10 years ago, and it's still true today.

My first football game as a sideline physician was in the fall of 2004. Going in, I felt I had all the training I needed. All of my board exams were successfully behind me; I was part of medical school faculty at the University of Michigan, with years of experience in the hospital setting; and I had taken care of patients along the entire spectrum of neurological disease.

I was, I thought, prepared.

I was so naïve.

Being new to watching a football game from my location on the sideline, I was immediately impressed with the speed of play, the nonstop complexity of the action, and the numerous, uncontrollable distractions.

Action happened on the field, players shuttled in and out of the lineup, multiple coaches yelled, fans cheered, and bands played, all while I was supposed to be practicing medicine. Indeed, it was a very strange place to be practicing medicine. Nothing about the sideline environment felt familiar. I immediately understood that providing medical care for athletes in a sporting environment would be a different, even difficult experience. I quickly developed a deep respect for the physicians and athletic trainers who came before me.

I also remember feeling a strange sense of disorientation at first. I knew sports well. I knew medicine well. But neither felt familiar here. Where was my quiet, controlled, distraction-free clinic room? Taking a step back in my mind, I took it all in, waiting for a neurological injury to occur, observing the players for any signs of brain dysfunction so that I could immediately perform a more detailed assessment, develop my opinion, and deliver care.

And yet when a linebacker came off the field, brought over to me with clear signs of brain injury—he was stumbling and incoherent—by the team's athletic trainer, I found myself pausing for a moment, not really believing what I saw. For the first time in my professional career, I could evaluate a patient for concussion immediately after a hit. Right off the bat, I was struck by how much the player reminded me of patients who were in the early stages of having a stroke. He favored one side of his body, appearing to be weak on the other. He couldn't answer my questions, because he didn't seem able to understand them. He was having a hard time following even simple directions. I was ready to call for the ambulance. The athletic trainer, who had been doing his job for a long time, told me to wait a minute or two and continue to observe the player. Within a few minutes, the player seemed to regain his physical coordination and mental coherence.

I was amazed to see brain pathology manifest and yet quickly resolve itself in a way I wasn't expecting. This was very different from everything I had learned as a neurologist. I was truly a stranger in a strange land.

I was used to thinking a certain way about concussion. My training and experience as a neurologist had given me only partial insight. Back then, I seldom saw concussions, because patients with these injuries were rarely referred to neurologists. When we did see concussions, it was usually several days after they occurred, and the circumstances were quiet, organized, and classically medical. I had never evaluated a patient only a few seconds after a collision, in that type of setting, with a concussion developing in front of me. It was scary, it was intriguing, and it challenged a lot of what I thought I knew about the injury.

The player indeed had a concussion, and as I evaluated him every day, I ultimately watched him fully recover. Just 24 hours after his injury, he showed very few symptoms and had a completely normal neurological examination. He sat out all football activities for two days, then returned back to activity gradually, and was playing full-contact football in practice nine days later. I learned something that first day on the sideline and in the week that followed that would change my mindset: Concussions have their own dynamic.

RESPECTING CONCUSSION'S COMPLEXITY

I now have learned something else from personal experience, having evaluated athletes on the sidelines and in locker rooms for over a decade: If you've seen one concussion . . . you've seen one concussion. Each situation is unique, and each injury its own challenge. Taking a simplified approach to concussion does our patients a huge disservice. Time and again, we hear about the new test that will help physicians, athletic trainers, and even non-medical staff, coaches, and parents to diagnose concussion. Again, I wish it were that simple. It just isn't.

Another factor to keep in mind with respect to problems diagnosing sports-related concussions is the nature of sports medicine itself. Classically, sports medicine has been largely based in orthopedics. More recently, primary care sports medicine has evolved to include caring for non-surgical orthopedic injuries as well as dealing with more standard primary care issues as they occur in athletes. The problem is that sports medicine, whether orthopedic or not, is steeped in a formulaic, protocol-based approach to medical care. Athletes and coaches are used to hearing that a certain degree of joint injury, for example, means a certain amount of time missed. Orthopedic injuries, by their nature, are easy to confirm with diagnostic tests. The examination techniques are straightforward, injury effects are relatively consistent, and the natural history of these injuries is fairly predictable. Thus a protocol approach works fine in these cases.

One of the main reasons concussions and long-term brain health have become such a public health concern in athletes is that sports medicine has, until very recently, taken this same approach to brain injury. Checklist medical histories, simple tests touted as diagnostic tools, and recommendations and protocols consistently applied from one injury to the next have dominated concussion care, each of these things ignoring one very obvious truth: The brain is very complex.

Our human brains are perhaps the most complex things in the universe. And we need to respect that fact.

Using a checklist of diagnostic criteria designed with ease in mind or relying on any one quick test on the sideline is not going to reliably diagnose concussion. A proper neurological assessment requires perspective, training, experience, and a good healthy dose of respect for the brain. It requires understanding how humans behave under different scenarios and how brain injury and disease present themselves across the wide variety of the human population. It requires getting to know your patients as complete individuals and understanding why they might be reacting as they are to what just happened during practice or a game.

The formulaic nature of sports medicine is one of the areas of concussion care that we must improve. The quality of diagnostic approach and management that athletes—especially our youngest athletes—receive varies widely. We can, and should, do better.

COMPARING AGAINST
A BASELINE

There are ways to best navigate the process of getting sound, thorough care for your youth athlete.

First, depending on competition level, age of the athlete, and resources, there may be a service available (or even mandated) referred to as *baseline testing*. Essentially, "baseline test" is a generic term for a formalized evaluation of brain function: cognitive or physical tests that are ideally administered and interpreted by a medical professional.

The concept of baseline testing is to get a snapshot of what the athlete's brain function looks like in an uninjured state. The test is typically done before the start of a season. A good baseline evaluation should also include gathering information from the athlete about any prior history of concussions, whether diagnosed or suspected. Additional medical history is also essential, including information on the presence of any other neurological disease, such as attention deficit hyperactivity disorder (ADHD), depression, anxiety, or migraine headache. Of course, any brain-affecting medications that the athlete is taking should also be noted.

These tests can vary widely in complexity and time requirements, but some of the most popular are computerized cognitive evaluations that last up to 45 minutes. Other tests can involve pencil and paper or more physical tasks. As an aside, I do not advocate for or against any one particular test. However, each baseline test is different, and the individuals administering and interpreting the tests should be well versed in the ones they use.

Before conducting any baseline test, the evaluator should be aware of whether the test being used is age appropriate. Unfortunately, not many testing mechanisms for athletes under age 12 have been well studied. That doesn't mean we shouldn't do baseline testing on our youngest athletes, but taking additional caution about the results and how they are used should be the rule.

A baseline test of any type may be useful when a concussion occurs. The same test that was administered to the athlete before (i.e., at baseline) should be given after the injury. Comparing the new results with the original ones serves as an extension of the physician's physical examination that can give insight as to the presence or absence of injury.

This comparison can also be useful in the post-diagnosis management of concussion.

There is one major caveat, however. Baseline testing, especially in the form of computerized neurocognitive tests, is more and more being used incorrectly throughout the United States. I would say that as I write this sentence in early 2016, baseline tests are more often used incorrectly than correctly here. In short, this is happening because many institutions have decided that these tests are all they need for a "concussion program." Despite warnings and legal statements from the companies that make some of the more popular tests that their tools "do not diagnose concussion," that still is exactly how they are used.

In the end, remember this one simple truth: Baseline testing is only as good as the medical professional using it.

As I have mentioned, there are several formats of baseline tests out there, and I urge further caution against those being promoted commercially. Concussion, as it turns out, has become a huge business!

More and more, school districts, sports leagues, and other institutions mandate baseline testing for all athletes as part of a formalized concussion or sports health protocol. Other organizations make it optional. Baseline testing is usually not covered by health insurance, but it can be cost-effective if a group of students or a school's worth of athletes all take the test.

It is important to not lose sight of the fact that baseline testing is only a means to gather potentially useful information.

It is not an insurance policy against an incorrect diagnosis, nor will it prevent long-term issues by themselves. Baseline tests are medical tests providing data that may—or may not—help a medical professional diagnose or manage a concussion.

FROM THE FIELD OF PLAY TO THE SIDELINE

Imagine you're with a youth athlete, and there has been an incident during the course of play or during a drill. The athlete runs into another player or into something hard like a goalpost or a lacrosse stick. Or maybe the athlete trips and falls awkwardly. Or maybe the athlete gets hit from behind and incurs a whiplash-mechanism injury to the neck. In any of these cases, the brain may have been jolted to a significant degree.

There are two routes by which a suspected concussion might come to light—one from the athlete and the other from someone around him or her: a coach, athletic trainer, parent, or teammate who witnessed the event itself or for another reason feels the athlete could be injured. The athlete could be displaying any of a number of signs of distress, including but not limited to confusion, head pain, neck pain, blurred vision, nausea, vomiting, or just not acting normally.

Remember, most concussions do not result in a loss of consciousness. So don't look for that as the sure sign a concussion has happened. Instead, the possibly concussed athlete may be uttering something along the lines of "I got my bell rung," "I got rocked," or "I saw stars."

In some cases, athletes who have experienced a significant blow are indeed knocked unconscious. When unconscious, some will also display an involuntary movement called *posturing*. These athletes will typically extend both arms out in front of them momentarily. Their wrists may also curl inward. This distinct reaction, lasting for a second or two, is a serious signal of a neurological disturbance of some kind.

Coaches, athletic trainers, athletes, and, yes, parents should know what to do from the very moment there is any suspicion of a concussion: The athlete must come out of the game or practice to get evaluated. There should be no tolerance for athletes' saying they are fine. There can be no shaking it off or pleading for more time to stay in the game.

Taking possibly concussed athletes out of play is more than a good sports medicine practice or a progressive coaching philosophy. It's now law, with all 50 states and the District of Columbia having passed legislation between 2009 and 2014 mandating that youth concussions be taken seriously.[1] Most states have specific laws, usually called Return to Play legislation, spelling out that athletes must leave play for proper evaluation if a concussion or traumatic brain injury (TBI) is suspected. The laws usually bar athletes from returning to play the same day the suspected concussion occurred. Many of the laws also spell out thresholds to be met before a concussed youth athlete can return to play, such as having an evaluation and subsequent written clearance to play from a medical professional.

Each state has its own set of particular points and language, but as a general rule, most Return to Play laws have the following features:

- If a concussion is suspected, the athlete must be removed from participation until they can be evaluated by a licensed healthcare provider (LHCP).
- If a concussion is diagnosed, the athlete is not to return to athletic participation for at least the remainder of the day on which the injury occurred.
- Once a concussion is diagnosed, the injured athlete cannot return to athletic participation until cleared to do so by a LHCP.
- Coaches, athletes, or both must receive some form of education about concussions.

A good place to check out the law in your area is at the Centers for Disease Control's website under its concussion policies area.[2]

Taking the time for an assessment and making sure the athlete stays out of play if potentially concussed are important for a number of reasons. Yes, the athlete's medical condition needs to be checked, but protection from getting another injury is also necessary if she or he is in a weakened or vulnerable state.

STEP ONE AFTER A SUSPECTED CONCUSSION

The injured athlete should be immediately evaluated by the school or club's athletic trainer, if one is available. Hopefully this is the case, as the athletic trainer is a critical part of starting a strong evaluation moments after a possible injury. If no trained medical personnel are present, it's always best to err on the side of caution. Parents and coaches should be prepared to respond to a potential injury, having a clear and communicated plan in place for assuring the activation of emergency medical services (EMS) when appropriate.

By now, most athletic trainers are trained in concussion protocols and likely will run the possibly injured player through an evaluation called the SCAT3 (Sports Concussion Assessment Tool, 3rd edition) or, in the case of a younger athlete, the Child-SCAT3. I was honored to be part of the group of experts that developed the SCAT3, the most recent update of the Sports Concussion Assessment Tool, released as a global standard in 2012. The SCAT3 is essentially a way to collect information about the athlete's brain function for use in the clinical decision-making process. Athletes are asked a series of questions that call for rating their sensations on a scale of 0 (no symptoms) to 6 (severe symptoms): Are you sensitive to light? What about sounds? Do you have a headache? Do you feel pressure in the head? Cognitive functioning is also tested, from immediate memory (such as giving the athlete a few words to remember, then asking him or her to repeat the sequence back) to orientation (checking whether the athlete knows the day of the week, time, and place). The SCAT3 can be used on the sidelines, in the training room, or in the physician's office. Note that the SCAT3 (and tools like it) is meant to be used by medical professionals. It is not meant to be a stand-alone diagnostic tool.

Having appropriate medical personnel, such as a certified athletic trainer, on the sidelines is a great way to increase the chances that this evaluation process will work well. Another asset is having an athletic trainer who knows the athletes personally, since that relationship can serve as a strong diagnostic aid. Such a person can answer questions like: Is the athlete acting differently from normal? Does he or she look different from normal? Insight into the athlete's personality and demeanor during normal times can provide a good index for comparison during a sideline evaluation for concussion.

Jason Hodges has served as an athletic trainer for USA Hockey's National Team Development Program for 17 years. He sees his role as an athletic trainer as a crucial link in protecting his youth hockey players on a daily basis. Hodges knows his players, and that gives him an advantage in times of injury.

"As an athletic trainer, I am the first line of defense for my athletes," Hodges says. "My sole purpose is the health and safety of the athletes. I am in the trenches with them every day, so I get to know them and their personalities. This relationship helps me as a medical provider if an athlete gets injured to know how they may handle an injury situation."

The tools to evaluate concussion on site are always improving. The SCAT, for example, has undergone three revisions over the past decade as medical research and feedback from sports physicians, athletic trainers, and athletic associations have provided additional depth of knowledge. New tools are being developed all the time, designed to help sport clinicians diagnose and manage concussion.

But remember my lesson that a sideline is a challenging and chaotic environment in which to conduct an evaluation. It is the exact opposite of a quiet, private space in a medical clinic. And keep in mind that even the best athletic trainers and doctors on the sidelines cannot see every play, or every player, so it's important for everybody to be vigilant and look out for player welfare.

Despite the best evaluations from a sideline athletic trainer or even a neurologist like myself, a concussion is not always detectable. Or the injury may not be detectable during the examination period. The symptoms of concussion can develop over hours, making an immediate protocol run-though a mere snapshot of what was occurring at the time, not a full picture of what could be developing later.

That's why taking an athlete with a suspected concussion out of play, whether from practice or a game, is such an important safeguard, and would be even if it weren't the law. It is especially critical that the sitting-out clause be followed for the youngest athletes. If there is reason enough to believe that athletes could be concussed, then there is reason enough to leave them out of play. The key to ensuring that this step is taken is having a strong protocol for communication from the medical evaluator on the sidelines to the coaches about whether or not an athlete is fit to play.

A CONCUSSION
IS DETECTED—WHAT'S NEXT?

The reality is that the majority of concussions do not require a trip to the emergency room. That being said, I always tell parents and coaches to err on the side of safety if there is ever any doubt. Sure signs that going to the ER is the best course of action include the following:

- a prolonged period of being unconscious after a hit (five minutes or longer)
- dramatically worsening symptoms of headache, vomiting, or increasing sleepiness.

Again, being conservative is the key. If you find it hard to keep the injured player's attention and carry on a conversation, it will make everybody more comfortable to seek urgent care from a medical provider.

As I've mentioned, many concussions don't produce dramatic symptoms or may not even produce a notable symptom for hours after a hit. In these cases, when concussion is suspected but not yet diagnosed, the best medicine is to be observant. It's a commonly held belief that when somebody hits his head hard enough to cause continued symptoms, he shouldn't go to sleep right away and should be woken up every hour. There's no hard and fast rule about this, but the idea is to use repeated evaluations to help rule out a more serious injury, namely, a bleeding episode inside of the skull. The most important thing to look for is the individual's level of consciousness. The person may be sleepy but should also be easily aroused to wakefulness. If there's any level of concern, activate emergency services immediately. The good news is, cases of bleeding in the skull are rare compared with concussions, and when they do occur, the declining consciousness of the patient is usually noted within the first couple of hours. Given the seriousness of this injury, I recommend four hours of frequent observation with a check at least every 15 minutes, after which time it's reasonable to let the person rest. That being said, it's always a good idea to be more careful than not, so it's definitely just as reasonable to sacrifice one night of sleep for extra assurance.

Even though most concussions don't require a trip to the ER, they should trigger a trip to a physician who has experience with concussion and who, if possible, knows the patient in question. Diagnosing a concussion is not easy and, as discussed earlier, cannot be done using a simple physical test, a computer test, or any type of checklist approach. Concussions are what we refer to as *clinical diagnoses*. They are diagnosed by a clinician who understands the complexity of brain function and can perform and interpret a comprehensive neurological evaluation. The clinician also is familiar with other conditions that either can mimic a concussion or frequently coexist with one and that cloud the picture.

The first step to concussion recovery is being properly diagnosed. Unfortunately, misdiagnoses of concussion are common, and becoming more common all the time. There is an assumption by many people, driven home daily by "conventional wisdom" and misinformation, that any time somebody experiences any neurological symptom after taking a blow to the head or body, the cause must be a concussion—especially if the person was playing a sport. While concussion should always be suspected in these cases, it is far from a given.

POSSIBLE, PROBABLE, AND DEFINITE CONCUSSIONS

Recently, the neurological community has begun clarifying concussion diagnoses by including a description of probability. I hear "You're either concussed or you're not" quite commonly in the media, usually from non-medical people. The problem is, that "concussed or not" line of thinking implies that every concussion is the same. If there were a simple confirmatory test that performed without fail and identified every, or almost every, concussion accurately, then yes, you could say that people are either concussed or not. It is true that technically, a concussion must exist or not, but we often do not know which is the case. So when we discuss the diagnosis with our patients or with colleagues, our inability to confirm the injury with an objective test means it is much better medical practice to frame the injury as a possible, probable, or definite concussion than to pretend we always have an unquestionable diagnosis.[3]

A *definite* concussion occurs when there is a clearly witnessed blow, or series of blows, that produces symptoms or physical findings that cannot reasonably be from any other cause. Examples include an obvious and immediate loss of consciousness following a helmet-to-helmet hit.

The term *probable* concussion should be used when there is a clearly witnessed blow, or series of blows, and a collection of neurological symptoms or findings that occur afterward that are probably from concussion but may be from some other cause. An example of a probable concussion would be a situation in which the presenting symptoms might be from concussion or might be from a headache disorder, such as migraine, or another brain disorder, such as ADHD. The key to this diagnosis is that even though the physician has identified other possible causes, concussion is still the most likely explanation.

Finally, a *possible* concussion is best described as a situation in which other possible explanations for symptoms or findings are more likely than concussion. In this case, clear alternative diagnoses should have been established. The term "possible concussion" also can be used when there is no clear physical insult and the onset of the injury is undetermined. This circumstance can occur easily in sports that include frequent collisions and a large number of players, such as football.

Aside from diagnostic accuracy, there is another important reason to use these terms to describe the certainty of a concussion diagnosis. It is commonly assumed that a concussion can always be diagnosed on the sidelines of a game or practice with a single evaluation if that evaluation is only complete enough. While concussions are often diagnosed with some degree of certainty on the sidelines, it is also common that a concussion cannot be diagnosed right away. A concussion might be suspected based on a particularly notable hit, even when the athlete has no symptoms or findings. It's also common that only minimal symptoms occur, such as a mild headache or neck discomfort. These symptoms occur frequently in sports, for many reasons, including dehydration, overheating, illness, or muscle strain. In these kinds of cases, it's often most accurate to describe the injury as a possible concussion.

Naturally, the degree of certainty of a concussion diagnosis can change over time. As with many things in neurology, the passage of time can be a very useful diagnostic test. Often, whether a concussion has or has not occurred is much clearer several hours after a hit, or even the next day. Don't be surprised if your athletic trainer or physician modifies the diagnosis as time goes on. Ultimately, the best perspective on how a concussion behaved and the best assessment of its cause come when the concussion is over.

Even though this approach to concussion terminology can help us better understand and describe the complexity of the diagnosis, I don't want you to get too caught up in the words. In the end, what your doctor provides as the specific diagnosis is only part of the story. The other part, which is much more important, is how the case is managed. Whether we say that you are probably concussed or possibly concussed doesn't matter as much as whether or not we treat you *as if* you are concussed.

MAKING ALL
THE RIGHT MOVES

So what does all this mean for you as an athlete? Simply this: If while participating in any sporting activity you experience a hit that would cause your brain to move quickly, a concussion should at least be suspected and you should be observed closely. If you show any signs of brain dysfunction, such as stumbling, a vacant stare, or difficulty communicating, you should be pulled from the game or practice. And you should not return to play until a trained medical professional can evaluate you in a comprehensive manner. (If you're a parent or someone else concerned with an athlete's care, I'm sure you can figure out what these recommendations mean for your own behavior.)

Once you've received a diagnosis of concussion, it's a great idea to become as informed as possible on what it means—not only its technical meaning, but also its implications for how you will be living in upcoming weeks and when you can return to your sport. Managing concussion and the return to participation is a complex medical job. Do not take it lightly. You should ask the doctor who diagnosed your concussion to explain how he or she came to that conclusion. Understanding how confident your doctor is in the diagnosis can help frame your expectations and map out the best road to recovery.

Even more, you should ask if the doctor considered any other possibilities. While this could be an uncomfortable question, most physicians will understand where it's coming from, especially with all of the media and public attention surrounding concussion. Those who can't answer the question or appear insulted to be asked likely don't have enough experience caring for patients with neurological conditions. And you definitely don't want to ignore any other medical issues that might be going on, even if they aren't related to the concussion per se.

Every week in my clinic, I hear stories from all points on the spectrum of treatment. One patient comes in after being told to jump right back into sports when "you feel like yourself again." The next one has been told to sit out a certain number of days regardless of how she's feeling. Then comes the inevitable patient who's been told to never play his sport again, that medical advice having been based only on the number of times he was diagnosed with concussion. Simplistic or predetermined plans like these make me question whether the caregiver understands the complexity of brain function and neurological injury.

For the best possible outcome, you want to be confident in your medical care provider's ability to identify all possible contributors to how you're feeling. Then, and only then, you can begin down the road to recovery.

REFERENCES

1. National Conference of State Legislatures. Traumatic brain injury legislation. July 28, 2014. http://www.ncsl.org/research/health/traumatic-brain-injury-legislation.aspx.
2. Centers for Disease Control and Prevention. Sports concussion policies and laws. http://www.cdc.gov/concussion/policies.html.
3. Giza C, Kutcher JS. Sports concussion diagnosis and management. *Continuum (Minneapolis, Minnesota)* 2014;20(6 Sports Neurology):1552–1569. doi:10.1212/01.CON.0000458974.78766.58.

Four

Life After a Diagnosis of Concussion

You've been diagnosed with a concussion. Now what?

At this point, it's natural if you have a few questions, and maybe some fears too. It's important to realize that the majority of concussions, up to 90 percent in some studies, produce symptoms for no more than a couple of weeks. It's important as well to understand that while the concussion you currently have might seem like the most urgent, most important thing that's going on in your life, you and your treating physician should also be looking at a bigger picture: A concussion is not only an injury to recover from. It's also an opportunity for your physician to evaluate your overall brain health by looking into your past, and for you both to carefully consider how to keep your brain healthy in the future.

THE FIRST FEW HOURS

Once a concussion has been identified and more serious injuries have been ruled out (see Chapter 3), the next step

67

is to look for any other ongoing medical conditions. For example, dehydration is common in athletics and should be addressed by having the concussed person drink plenty of fluids—preferably water or appropriate sports drinks. Neck strain, sleep disturbances, and headaches are also common for reasons other than concussion. In essence, an athlete with a concussion should not be assumed to have only a concussion.

As for the concussion itself, the first few hours are mainly about symptom control. Quite often, a concussion will produce not only headache but also sensitivity to light and sound, making it difficult to stay in a sports environment. Think of the hectic environment of a game or practice. Coaches yelling, whistles blowing, players running and cutting, objects flying through the air, and bright light from the sun or stadium lights are all part of the playing conditions for athletes. Then throw in some thumping, blaring music over the top of that. It usually feels better for the concussed athlete to go into the locker room or a quiet indoor space, where the sensory environment can be better controlled. This should only happen, however, if a responsible adult is present to continue observation. A recently concussed person should not be left alone for the first few hours after the injury.

Other common symptoms include nausea and clumsiness. It's fine to use over-the-counter anti-nausea treatments. Patients should be made as comfortable as possible and should not be expected to perform any physical or mental task. Confusion and memory difficulties may limit the ability to do even simple tasks, and the injured person should not drive or use any motorized equipment.

In those first few hours, there will likely be an urge to give the concussed athlete a medication to treat their headache. Acetaminophen-based pain relief medication (like Tylenol) can be used, but over-the-counter anti-inflammatory medications such as ibuprofen (Motrin) and naproxen (Aleve) should be avoided at least for the first 24 hours. The latter medications can promote bleeding, so if there is a bleed inside the skull, they may make it worse.

It's also important in the first several hours for the patient to keep hydrated and take in some calories. I prefer at this stage for the patient to eat foods that aren't spicy or otherwise hard on the stomach. Simple carbohydrates, proteins, and a well-balanced nutrient load are your best bets. Athletic recovery shakes often fit the bill nicely.

ACUTE REST PHASE

"REST!" has been the long-standing mantra of concussion management. The simple and widely used version of this advice is to rest until you no longer have symptoms. This idea has been promoted mainly because symptoms were long felt to be the only way to identify the presence of a concussion. However, it is possible to not have any symptoms and still be injured. It is also possible to have symptoms several days after a hit that are not from the concussion itself.

Overall, the first 24–48 hours after the injury continue to be about patient comfort. I use the term *acute rest* to describe this phase. The overall idea is to do very little other than what physicians call "activities of daily living." In other words, I want patients to go out of their way to do less than normal. Probably, the patient will feel bad enough to not want to do much anyway, so the advice "Don't do anything" is usually welcomed.

The acute rest phase is also the best time to look ahead at the next week or two and identify any upcoming academic, athletic, or social responsibilities that may need to be rescheduled. Much like the rest of concussion management, this phase can vary in duration. On average, it will last one to three days, but it can be longer. I don't use a predetermined number of days for this phase of recovery. I find the patient's own symptoms and tolerance for doing things to be the best guide for how long it should last. When patients feel like participating in life, I let them do so.

A very common suggestion at this point is to avoid "screen time," such as watching television, using computers or tablets, gaming, and even texting. There's no hard scientific basis for this recommendation. Patients are often told that they should not do these things to avoid making their injury worse. While these activities might make a headache worse or produce an increased sense of mental fogginess, it's hard to imagine from a neuroscience perspective that the injury itself will get worse as a result. (It may be possible, if taken to extremes, for any of these activities to do further damage.) In general, my advice to patients is to avoid those things that make you feel significantly worse, but if you aren't overly troubled while texting or surfing the Web, then go ahead. You may just want to do so in small, bite-size chunks.

At the same time that we recommend doing very little, we must realize that significantly isolating a concussed person may produce unintentional negative effects. When somebody stays at home instead of being at school and misses the social interaction of being around friends or teammates, there is a natural tendency to feel alone. It is also very common for patients to feel depressed during the first few days of a concussion. This feeling is a common direct effect of the injury itself. Sometimes, however, the depression is obviously happening because the patient has been removed from regular life and is missing being part of a group.

During the acute rest phase, it's important to be supportive and encouraging. Let the patient go to school—if he feels like it—but also be prepared with backup plans if things do not go well there. Leaving a particular class early, or even going home from school early, is certainly an option. Don't let the patient work out in any significant way or dive into tough academic work at home. But also don't turn the patient into a mushroom . . . unless that's all he can handle.

It's reasonable to use medication for headache during the acute rest phase, most notably over-the-counter anti-inflammatory medications. These can be used either as needed for headache, up to twice a day, or in a scheduled fashion. But remember, headache medicine of this kind should be avoided in the first 24 hours of a suspected concussion. And even if you are just using an over-the counter medication, it's important to let your doctor know you're doing so.

Similarly, sleep aids, such as melatonin, can be very helpful in the right situation. Sleep is quite commonly disturbed by concussion, with some patients having a hard time falling asleep, some waking frequently, and some doing both. It's also common for individuals recovering from a concussion to sleep during the day, even if they're staying asleep for a good chunk of the night. This happens because not all sleep is created equal. Just because sleep occurred does not mean it was enough to promote rest and healing. To be restorative, sleep needs to be of the right quality and the correct amount.

Any noticeable change in sleep pattern should be considered significant and reported to your doctor. During the acute rest phase, I typically advise patients to let their brain set the clock and sleep when they're tired.

Nausea can also be treated symptomatically in this phase, especially if it is limiting the patient's ability to eat or stay hydrated. To help support the brain's recovery, it's very important both to keep up with caloric needs and to take in enough fluids. My usual advice is to ask patients to drink at least one 12-ounce glass of water three times a day, even if they're not thirsty.

When using any medication or supplement, whether for headache, sleep, nausea, or anything else, it's important not to let the effects of these interventions cloud the true picture of recovery. As we continue to monitor improvement, we want to get the best possible sense of what symptoms the injury is still producing. This will become even more important a little further into the recovery process.

After a few days, most patients don't mind going about some the activities of daily life, and they should be encouraged to do so. This development is a sign that recovery is on the right track and should trigger a subtle but important change in the approach to the injury. The patient is now ready to enter the *relative rest* phase of recovery.

RELATIVE REST PHASE

The initial period of acute rest will naturally transition into the relative rest phase, when the concussion is still producing symptoms but the injured person can tolerate simple life activities without too much difficulty. During this phase, it is important to continue to avoid extremes of cognitive and physical exertion. It's also important to avoid extremes of rest and isolation.

At this point, it's worthwhile to pause in your reading and do a simple thought experiment. Take the average person, uninjured and in good health, and imagine telling her to do nothing for 14 days. No school, no work, no physical or social activity. Essentially, you are telling her check out of life for two weeks.

How do you think that average person would feel by the end of that period of imposed isolation?

Depending on the individual, she will feel anywhere from a little bit to a lot different from her normal state. Her sleep patterns will change, and her energy levels will be different. Some people will get just a little antsy, while others may become significantly more restless, to the point that it interferes with their ability to be productive. Some people will start to feel foggy or "out of it." Many will start to get headaches. Mood problems such as depression, attention issues such as ADHD, migraine headaches—really, any brain problem—can potentially get fuel to become more problematic under these circumstances.

You can see why the "REST!" approach to managing concussion can end up confusing matters. Rest is the very thing we tell our patients to do when they're diagnosed with concussion—and yet rest on its own can eventually produce symptoms that look a lot like those of concussion!

The longer a concussed person does nothing, the more likely these various issues will start to happen, and the more complicated true concussion recovery may become. In some people, this may open the door to another problem, post-concussion syndrome (which we will discuss in Chapter 5). This clinical nuance is one of the more challenging aspects of concussion care and among the many reasons no cookbook approach to managing the injury will work for everybody.

In the relative rest phase, it's important that the patient get moving and active, both physically and cognitively. The trick is to not do too much. Medications should be limited as much as possible, to help the doctor judge recovery and improvement. While contact sports should still be avoided, it is reasonable for the patient to start working out under a physician's guidance. A doctor who has experience not only with concussion and other brain injuries but with the entire spectrum of brain function and disease is best at managing this phase of recovery.

The relative rest phase typically lasts a few days, more or less. It can be identified as coming to an end when the patient is able to tolerate a full day of school or work without any notable symptoms.

Understanding when this phase is over is an inexact science and requires years of experience and a comprehensive approach to the patient's care. One useful tool is *observed exertion*. A patient who is able to tolerate very simple physical exertion, like working out on a stationary bike, without developing any significant symptoms or examination findings is likely coming to the end of the relative rest phase. The person is then ready to begin the directed return to participation in sports typically enacted during the *gradual exertion* phase.

GRADUAL EXERTION PHASE

The gradual exertion phase of recovery is often misunderstood. The idea is that once patients are able to tolerate regular life, they should be put through a series of challenges designed to expose the potentially still-injured brain to increasing levels of physical and cognitive exertion. These challenges are not designed to test athletes' ability to tolerate sporting activities or to see if they are athletically ready to go back to their sports. Rather, this process is essentially a form of diagnostic testing that gives the physician insight into whether the injury is still present.

This approach stems from still another important realization: A brain can be injured and not produce any symptoms or clinical effect at all. Therefore our job as concussion physicians is not to determine when somebody is feeling better but to determine when the injury itself is over. By exposing the brain to these increasing challenges, we are lowering the threshold for symptom production and so giving the brain the opportunity to "let us know" whether it is still injured.

But here's yet another problem: Individuals who perform a physical challenge after being inactive for a few days, whether they were injured or not, have the potential to experience symptoms just because they are working out again. This is especially true for young, physically active people. And the longer they've been inactive, the stronger the effect.

Let's say you're in a healthy, normal, and uninjured state and I ask you to ride a stationary bike to get your heart rate up into the 130s for 20 minutes. You might expect to have some feelings of lightheadedness or maybe a subtle sensation of pressure in your head. These same feelings are commonly misread as signs of the persistence of injury in a concussed person.

At the same time, there are definitely symptoms that can be a clue that somebody is still suffering from a concussion. Telling the difference between symptoms due to a temporary physiological condition (such as that produced by working out) and those due to injury or disease is one of the core elements of providing the best possible concussion care. The importance of distinguishing between these situations is yet another reason to seek the care and advice of a physician who is experienced in evaluating the full spectrum of neurological conditions.

Given that symptoms that can occur with or without concussion may arise as somebody progresses through the graduated exertion process, it's good to keep some general thoughts in mind. I like to sort any symptom that's being considered, such as headache, nausea, or light sensitivity, into one of three levels of concern:

Level I—Underneath the surface: These are symptoms you notice only when you stop and think about how you're feeling. Even then, sometimes it's hard to tell if

they're present or not. In my experience, continuing
an exertion task with Level 1 symptoms is perfectly
reasonable and safe.

Level 2—In the background: These symptoms are
strong enough to be present throughout the task at
hand but not bad enough to interfere with it. When
experiencing this level of symptom, it can still be OK
to continue, though it's best to proceed with caution.

Level 3—In your face: These symptoms make it difficult to keep doing the exertional task. They're bad
enough that you can't stop thinking about how you
feel. At Level 3, it's best either to stop the exertion or
to back it way down.

This is just a general framework. If you're a patient, I don't
want you to overthink every symptom that you feel. In the end,
if you're not comfortable or if you're exerting yourself when you
don't have a clinician directly observing your activity, I always
say to err on the side of being conservative. It is better to back
an exertion down or stop than to push through any particular
symptom.

During exertion testing, it's important to let your physician
know about any and every symptom you experience during or
after each level of exertion. An exertion challenge doesn't end
with the activity itself but only after enough time has passed to

allow symptoms to occur. Typically this is 24 hours, but the amount can vary from case to case.

If you perform an exertion challenge at one level and do well, meaning you certainly have not experienced any Level 3 symptoms and likely none at Level 2 either, and you still feel good roughly 24 hours later, then we typically let you go to the next level until you are cleared for full participation.

I can guess what you are now pondering: Given that certain symptoms can be concussion related or not, is it possible to have one best protocol governing return to participation in your sport?

Like most parts of concussion diagnosis and management, there should be a standard *approach* to this phase of recovery, but not a standard protocol. There is no one exact prescription. You may find some protocols that state, "Do this exact exertion for this amount of time," but this reflects an unsophisticated understanding of the human brain. Each situation depends on so many factors: the age of the patient, the sport (or sports) the person plays, the presence of other medical conditions, and more.

So it's best that the process of returning to participation be dynamic and flexible. It should rely not on some rigid and universal equation but rather on frequent and meaningful observation, re-evaluation, and guidance from an experienced clinician.

THE BRAIN PROCESS

Given these parameters, however, we can at least describe a basic framework that should be followed for exertional challenges. Years ago, I began referring to this as the BRAIN process. Here's what you would go through as an injured patient:

Bike (B): This first stage is all about introducing simple cardiovascular exertion in a way that is as boring as possible. We're not starting this way to punish you! We take this approach because we want the brain to experience little more than a mild, sustained increase in heart rate and blood pressure and a simple shift in your body's energy requirements. Our basic recommendation for this stage is to use a stationary bike (hence the "B") to provide enough exertion to increase pulse and breathing rates within a comfortable zone. A direct measure of heart rate may help guide this process, but since everybody is going to be in different states of conditioning, it's hard to have one target rate that fits everyone. I find that the best advice is to exert yourself to a level that makes you feel like you're working, but that would give you no trouble if you were having a normal conversation with somebody standing next to you.

You should continue this level of exertion for at least 20 minutes, up to 30 minutes maximum. Again, it might be

completely normal to feel some sensations of lightheadedness or mild pressure in the head. These feelings don't necessarily mean you need to stop. Remember the three levels
of symptoms outlined above: underneath the surface, in the
background, and in your face.

Run (R): This stage is designed to add simple movement to
what the brain is experiencing. This is best done on a tread-
mill; it can also be done on an elliptical machine or similar
device. The main idea is for you to do simple, repetitive move-
ments without worrying about what's going on around you.
Mild interval training can also be introduced at this stage.
While the majority of the exertion at this stage should be at a
nice sustained level as in the Bike stage, the exertion level can
be increased a little bit for 30–45 seconds at a time, two or
three times, during a 30-minute total workout.

Agility (A): This is the most complicated stage and the one
with the most variability from sport to sport and athlete to
athlete. At the core of this stage is the addition of complex,
quick maneuvers that move you around in space in different
ways, giving your brain a lot more to deal with. This stage is
also designed to include more interval-type exertions than in
the Run stage. Drills done in this stage can be standard gym
exercises, such as lunges, chops, and burpees, or they can be
sport specific. The idea is still to do an exertion that is at least
30 minutes long, but it's a good idea to go a little longer if
you can.

It's a really good thing for the physician to tailor the agility drills used in this stage to match what sport (or sports) you play. It's also worth paying attention to the environment in which the exertion takes place. Now would be a good opportunity to introduce a complex environment that includes a lot of activity and sound, such as a busy training facility.

"In Red" (I): This stage is named after the practice of putting the athlete into practice in a red jersey, which signifies that you're not to be hit or otherwise experience purposeful contact. (I know, this letter's a bit of a stretch, but I couldn't think of better "I" term that would let me spell BRAIN.) This stage is really about two things. First, it allows you to experience a full-duration practice with all of its sights, sounds, emotions, commotion, and activity. This will likely be the longest period of continuous exposure to exertion in any of the stages. Remember, the circumstances and the nature of the exertion will also depend on your specific sport. The second, and more critical, reason for this stage is to begin to expose you to the *cognitive load* required to play your sport.

The cognitive load of a sport consists of all the mental tasks that it takes to actually play it. Think about some of the more standard practice drills for your sport. Now think about how those are different from actually playing in a game or match. In a game, there's a lot more going on around you, more things to worry about. There are more complicated decisions to make and things to react to. You may need to take into account many more players around you than in a practice drill. These all contribute to your sport's cognitive load.

Some sports have a moderate amount of difference between doing drills and being in a game. Football is one of these. Plays in football last, on average, around 6.5 seconds, and practice drills are pretty similar in duration. But in a sport like ice hockey there's a tremendous gap between doing drills and playing in a game, because of the sport's continuous action, speed, and complex environment. (Sorry, football coaches!)

So when considering the "In Red" stage, it's good to think about the particular sport in question. For some sports, it may be better to address this stage in smaller, bite-size pieces. Start with interacting and playing with one teammate. Then add another, even several, and progress in that manner. Not every sport requires this approach, but for any sport it's essential to think about the potential difficulties of going from the isolated drills of the Agility stage to a complex game environment.

The final thing to consider during this stage is introducing some well-controlled and minimal contact. Physical sports such as football, men's lacrosse, or ice hockey will always involve some level of contact. I prefer to have the first contact my patients experience after concussion not be in a game. We do this in our clinic if we can, as part of our dynamic evaluation, but it can also take place in practice. I recommend this first contact occur only under the direct supervision of an experienced concussion clinician. And I want to emphasize that contact should start small and build up gradually. Do *not* go in full speed.

No Restrictions (N): Having gone through the four stages above, you're ready to return to play. Remember, this entire graduated return to participation is not just a series of steps designed to see if you are in shape or if your skills are up to game quality. This process is about giving your physician the best possible information with which to make the determination that your injury is over. In this final stage, your physician should carefully consider the entire injury again—from start to finish. Only after your physician has given you clearance should you return to playing a sport with any contact risk.

NOW WHAT?

Your concussion is over and your life should be back to normal. You may now find yourself wondering: What does this episode mean for the future? Will it be easier to get concussed again? Would the next one be worse? If it occurs, will I need to retire from sports? How many concussions is too many? Is there a number that will mean I'm in trouble?

Welcome to being normal, because these are all very common questions, asked by athletes at all levels!

To start, no number of concussions is an absolute, stand-alone determinant of when to retire. One, three, even 10 concussions . . . there is no magic number. And there are a few reasons why not.

First, as you've likely already gathered, each injury is different. So just saying you've had, say, three concussions doesn't really tell much of the story. To figure out the implications of your past concussions for your athletic future, we would need to talk about each injury specifically and in detail. Why and how did the injury occur? What was the actual force? How sensitive are you to getting symptoms? What were your symptoms like, and how long did they last? The variability in all of these things is just too great for a simple, hard number of concussions to mean much at all.

Second, while concussion is an important injury that needs to be taken very seriously, what matters most is the lifetime health of your brain. So it's important to put each concussion into this larger perspective. A comprehensive neurological evaluation and management plan should include not only the most recent injury you recovered from but also what happened to you further back in the past and what your plans are for the future. The number of diagnosed concussions alone cannot address these issues.

As for your concerns about what your concussion means for the likelihood and severity of future concussions, many of the statements you may hear about these issues fall into the category of oversimplifications or myths. It's repeated a lot that one concussion makes it easier to get another. That may be true for some individuals, especially those who had a complicated course of recovery from concussion. However, there is no good published data that truly speaks to this question. My clinical experience is that the vast majority of my patients do not have a decrease in their threshold for being injured or experiencing symptoms following a concussion, as long as the injury was identified early and appropriately managed.

Another popular assumption is that the next concussion will most likely be worse, in some way, than the previous one. Again, in my experience, this is not a typical pattern. Some patients may have worse symptoms if they get hit again before recovering from their concussion, but if a concussion is indeed over, the severity of the next concussion typically isn't predictable at all.

That said, while it may be rare for the threshold for incurring a concussion to decrease and for concussions to become increasingly severe over the course of a history of concussions, these phenomena do become very important to look for when considering whether it is time to retire from contact sports. However, the most important reason to retire from or limit exposure to contact sports is to preserve your long-term brain health. It's critically important that your physician have the training and experience to evaluate overall brain function and put it into the perspective of your entire life. For these greater overall considerations, it's not the concussions themselves that matter nearly as much as how your brain is functioning between the concussions.

Overall, it's important to know that a lowered concussion threshold and increased concussion severity can happen once someone has had one or more concussions, just not as often as people might think, and that if they do happen to you, the best thing may indeed be to retire from contact sports. The key to understanding if these circumstances apply to you is a very carefully done, thorough neurological evaluation. Deciding to retire from sport should be an informed decision, with the patient, doctor, and the patient's loved ones all playing a role in the discussion.

FIVE

POST-CONCUSSION SYNDROME AND SECOND-IMPACT SYNDROME

L et me take you through a hypothetical case.

A 16-year-old soccer player, whom I will to refer to as Anna, has come to my clinic because she isn't recovering from a concussion that occurred while she was in a game. It's been three months since the incident, which happened when she went up to play the ball in the air and an opponent accidentally elbowed her on the side of the head. The blow threw her off balance and she landed on her back, with the momentum causing the back of her head to strike the ground.

This sequence happened very fast and now is kind of a blur in Anna's memory, but she doesn't recall feeling any symptoms right away. She was able to get to her feet, still feeling a little unsteady, and continued to play. The play occurred early in the second half, and Anna played the rest of the game without a break. With about 10 minutes to go, she felt the start of a dull, nagging headache and noticed that she was a little bit behind the play.

After the game, she felt more tired than usual, went home, and went to bed earlier than she typically does. Her sleep was choppy at best, and she was waking up every 90 minutes or so. When she got up the next morning, she felt slow and lethargic—she says it was like somebody had "wrung me out like a sponge." She had a dull and constant headache, located between and just above her eyes.

Over the next seven days, Anna essentially stayed in her room. At the advice of her primary care doctor, she stayed home from school and didn't participate in any soccer or social activities. She also avoided her computer and cell phone, trying to help her brain rest.

Day by day, Anna's headache gradually began to improve, and her "fog" began to lift. Her sleep, however, continued to be erratic, and it is still a major problem. She falls asleep easily enough and sometimes naps during the day, but she has a hard time staying asleep and typically wakes up for good very early.

On the fourth day after her injury, Anna had tried to go to school, but she found that the lights and sounds made her head hurt worse. She left early, went back home, and continued to rest as much as she could.

On her seventh day home, which marked the one-week anniversary of her injury, Anna reported continued lingering symptoms of headache and light sensitivity. Even so, because she missed her soccer team, she decided to go watch them play in a game. She felt pretty well overall, even passing the ball back and forth on the sidelines with her friends during the 15-minute halftime break. But she also noted that the sun bothered her, and as the game went on she felt more "drained." Anna remembers very clearly feeling confused about what she should do: She wanted to stay and support her team but also wanted to be back home on the couch. In the end, she left the game during the second half.

Anna tried to go to school again the next week, despite not feeling 100 percent, but had the same results as before. She again had to leave early because of her sensitivities to light and sound. To this point, the only physical activity she had experienced since her injury diagnosis, other than her brief interaction with her teammates, was walking from one place to another. She hadn't been doing her typical chores around the house, and every time she walked more than a few paces, she noticed an increasing sensation of head pressure.

This pattern continued for the next two weeks without significant change, and now she sits in my clinic room, clearly withdrawn and sleepy, yawning frequently.

Anna and her mom can't understand why this concussion is so different from her only other diagnosed concussion, two years ago. That concussion lasted only four days or so. They are also concerned because Anna is scheduled to attend a Division II college soccer camp in three weeks. The college hosting the camp is where she wants to go to school and also where she would like to continue her soccer career . . . if she can.

A physician told Anna that this concussion is obviously worse than the last one and that this trend does not bode well for the future. Anna and her mom were also told that the next concussion would likely be even worse and could even lead to permanent changes in her brain function.

Anna admits this concussion has scared her and she now worries about never being able to play soccer again. She wants to keep playing, but is starting to realize that this injury could spell the end of her career. She is also concerned that she is destined to have headaches and fatigue for the rest of her life. Anna admits that her thinking isn't right either: She's forgetting things, even simple things that used to be easy to recall, and it is hard for her to do any academic activity for more than a few minutes at a time. Her grades are starting to fall. In many ways, her life is slipping away from her.

Unfortunately, this is an all-too-common story where concussion is concerned.

What's going on? Why is this concussion so much worse than Anna's previous one?

It turns out that the answer in this case, as in the majority of cases like it, is that Anna is not concussed at all. Not anymore, at least. While the original injury most likely was concussion, she is now suffering from post-concussion syndrome (PCS).

CLARIFYING AN ELUSIVE
MEDICAL SYNDROME

As a rule, whenever the word *syndrome* is used in the medical world, it's a good idea to be cautious. Often the specific information being discussed will be complex and ambiguous. Even the word itself should be a clue, as "syndrome" is derived from the Greek word for correlation, implying an association. The term is used to describe a pattern or collection of symptoms or findings that do not come from one single cause.

Post-concussion syndrome is an excellent example of this concept. The symptoms experienced in PCS are all results of the brain's producing a clinical effect when it's generally under duress, regardless of what the cause of duress is. Typical symptoms of PCS include:

- headaches
- fatigue
- depression
- neck pain
- "foggy thinking"
- sleep difficulties
- poor memory

But there can be many other symptoms as well. And none of them relate specifically to just one cause. In essence, any aspect of brain function can be affected in PCS. So like the good syndrome it is, PCS should be thought of not as one thing affecting the brain, but rather as a collection of things that may affect the brain, either alone or in different combinations, to produce the same end effects.

Now that we've covered what *syndrome* means, let's consider the remaining part of the term. *Post-concussion* means exactly what it sounds like: PCS occurs *after* the concussion is over. Putting the concepts of "post-concussion" and "syndrome" together, we can describe PCS clearly as a collection of neurological symptoms that occur in response to a concussion but are not caused directly by the concussion itself.

It can be difficult to tell concussion and PCS apart, because they involve similar symptoms. Making things a little more difficult, it is quite possible for somebody to still be experiencing symptoms from the concussion when the symptoms of PCS begin to develop. Since the symptoms of concussion and PCS are similar and often overlap in time, the outward appearance may be of a patient suffering from one long concussion. But the term "post-concussion syndrome" is not used to describe a longer-than-usual concussion. The concussion may have been the inciting event—the thing that opened the door for PCS to walk through—but the two diagnoses should not be confused for each other.

Think of the famous athletes you've heard about, or perhaps people you know, who had to sit out months at a time from their regular lives, or even whole seasons in the case of athletes, because of a "concussion." Some athletes may even have retired from their sports because of continued symptoms. The thing is, they most likely were no longer concussed. In most cases, they had PCS.

I'm not insisting on the distinction between concussion and PCS just to make an academic point. Despite the inherent difficulties in telling them apart, they are very different things with very different treatments. As both awareness of and concern over concussion have grown, an increasing proportion of patients have been stuck in a long PCS because they were being treated, incorrectly, for concussion. So telling the difference between them is critical.

THE IMPORTANCE OF TAKING A HISTORY

When physicians evaluate patients for concussion and PCS, the approach must be careful, critical, and comprehensive. As you now understand, there isn't a clear, objective, or absolute confirmatory test for concussion. What physicians do have is the ability to complete a thorough neurological history and examination. We can use various tools to augment or improve our examinations, but in the end, we put all of the information together to form a medical opinion that is often nuanced and that may evolve over time.

One common approach that you may have run into is one that frequently falls short: making the diagnosis solely based on the amount of time since the concussion happened. Some clinicians might use an arbitrary cutoff date, like four weeks or three months, to assign a diagnosis of PCS. While most concussions should be over at four weeks, this certainly isn't always the case. A clinician who behaves in this manner likely considers PCS and concussion to be the same thing or is treating PCS simply as a "long concussion."

Another common reason for misdiagnosis stems from clinicians' relying on symptom checklists for a neurological history. These checklists typically consist of a set of symptoms, each with a numerical scale (typically from 0 to 6) on which patients rank the intensity with which they are experiencing the symptom. Often, patients will fill out the checklist before meeting with the doctor. Symptom checklists are commonly used in concussion diagnosis and management, either as stand-alone tools or as a portion of a large tool like the SCAT3. There is no doubt that taking a systematic approach to asking patients about potential symptoms is important. However, there is a big difference between extracting good clinical information from a patient and simply running through a checklist.

When physicians are taught to take a neurological history, they are told to start with broad questions and become more focused as they proceed. The first question might simply be, for example, "What symptoms are bothering you?"

Every symptom that the patient mentions is then fleshed out in greater detail. The only way to separate out and fully understand each symptom is by asking a progression of questions—things like:

"When did it start?"
"Is it constant?"
"What makes it worse or better?"
"What other symptoms come with it?"
"Is it improving, getting worse, or staying the same?"

These are just a few of the questions required to help understand a single symptom. There are many, many, more. When the answers to all the questions about symptoms are taken together, they give the fullest, clearest overall clinical picture.

So you can imagine that if you went to a doctor with "only" three or four symptoms, getting a proper history could take a while! Actually, it *should* take some time to discuss everything with your doctor. If a symptom is important enough to help the physician make a diagnosis or dictate management, it will take more, and more precise, questions to zero in on the relevant details.

Compare this approach with having a patient rate a headache on a scale from 0 to 6. That may not a bad place to start, but it leaves a lot left to be uncovered. This is one of the reasons I tell clinicians that if you're evaluating patients with concussion (or PCS or another brain disorder) and your schedule shows that you're seeing more than one patient an hour, you're likely doing it wrong.

THE TROUBLE WITH CHECKLISTS

Research studies have shown symptom checklists to be sensitive for concussion screening. That doesn't mean that they're good for clinical care. I hate to say this, but in the real clinical environment (as opposed to the artificial, controlled world of research), they may do more overall harm than good. There are three main reasons why.

First, symptom checklists are often used as crutches or shortcuts around taking a good neurological history. The clinician stops thinking and doesn't ask the important follow-up questions that would help the patient tremendously in the long run.

Second, filling out a symptom checklist has an interesting effect on some people, especially if they are asked to fill one out frequently (like on a daily basis). I had a recent patient who, right at the start of the visit, gave me an interesting answer to my opening question, "What brings you to see me today?" She replied with, "I think I'm stuck between numbers." The patient had become so fixated on the numbers listed as options on the checklist that she forgot what her "normal" condition was. This kind of reaction to checklists can give some people a heightened sense of anxiety and actually propagate the perception of symptoms.

The third reason is simple: People are unique, meaning one person's "3" can be another person's "1" or "6." Some patients, when asked to rate their pain on a numeric scale of 1 to 10, with 10 being the highest level of pain they could possibly imagine, sit there very comfortably with a normal heart rate and breathing rate, look you in the eye, and say "10." No matter how many times you explain things, they insist they are in the worst pain imaginable.

How is that possible? Are they lying? No, they're not, at least not necessarily. There is a difference between "pain itself" and the "perception" of pain. Experiencing any sensation, from any sensory organ, involves two tightly coupled processes. The first is getting information from the environment using sensory receptors, whether on your tongue, in your nose, on your skin, or elsewhere—including the receptors in your body that send your brain signals about your internal environment. The second process involves how the brain processes and interprets that information to produce a perception of that sensation. In this way, what we experience in our lives is just as much about what we do with the signals we get as it is about the signals themselves. So patients who are "objectively" not in much pain can still perceive themselves as suffering greatly.

Something similar goes for taking and interpreting a neurological history. The absolute information extracted from the patient, such as the number of headaches, duration of episodes of dizziness, or the perception of foggy thinking or fatigue, is important, without question. But it is only the first part of the story. The second part is putting it all together by noticing *how* the information is given, evaluating the context of this episode in the person's life, and determining how the person in front of you tends to experience the world.

Try doing that with a checklist.

So taking a good neurological history is essential for the physician. If you're the injured person, on the other hand, you can help by giving a good history. Be thoughtful and complete with your answers, but let your interviewer guide the process. At the same time, it's a great idea to make a list of your concerns ahead of meeting with your physician, to make sure they are all covered in appropriate detail.

Once we have a thorough history, how does that help us decide between concussion and PCS?

As a very general rule, concussion symptoms tend to resolve in a linear fashion. Day by day there should be progressive, though sometimes slow, improvement. When there are significant or dramatic increases in concussion symptoms, they're usually due to an additional event, such as a few days of tough academic work or going back to sports too soon. Patients who are resting appropriately and avoiding extremes of exertion tend to get better at a constant rate until they are more or less back to themselves.

The timing of PCS symptoms, on the other hand, is generally a bit more unpredictable. They tend to vary more frequently and sometimes unpredictably. There's also usually a sense that the more somebody with PCS rests, the more the symptoms stay the same—or even get worse. In many cases, a clear period of improvement as the concussion is healing is followed by a plateau—and that's a hint that another process is coming into play.

A thorough neurological history will help your physician consider all of the potential causes of your symptoms and possibly point to PCS as the cause. But the history is just the first essential step of establishing (or ruling out) a PCS diagnosis. The next one is the physical examination.

DYNAMIC PHYSICAL EVALUATIONS

It's pretty standard for a doctor or any healthcare provider to do a physical examination when the patient is in a state of relative rest, typically sitting on a clinic examination table in a calm, quiet room. The neurological examination is no different. Neurologists are trained to do a very detailed and specific physical examination that classically is performed while the patient is in a state of relative calm and rest.

Many things that clinicians ask you to do during a physical examination are designed to have a particular body part perform some function. For example, by listening to your lungs while you breathe deeply, your doctor is able to consider different aspects of your lung function and look for signs that indicate normal or abnormal function. Using function to inform a physical examination is an incredibly important concept. How does a particular examination finding change when the physician asks the patient to perform a task? The answer can be very enlightening.

This is also true of the neurological examination, of course. Your neurologist might ask you to balance on one foot, for example, to examine a particular neurological function. How you do this task gives him or her information about a particular piece of the nervous system. When it comes to brain function, however, we sometimes need to have the patient do something a bit more dynamic than just standing on one foot. Many of the symptoms and associated examination findings of PCS can best be brought out by certain types of complex physical activities. Other symptoms of PCS might actually be helped by particular tasks. It all depends on the patient and their situation.

For example, a patient who is experiencing foggy thinking or dizziness one month after a concussion might actually feel better after a 20-minute ride on a stationary bike at a moderate level of exertion. She might get a short bout of increased dizziness or a sensation of head pressure, but this often subsides quickly.

Asking a patient to perform a series of complex physical maneuvers that have her spinning or jumping while also performing cognitive tasks at different degrees of exertion or difficulty can help with something altogether different. It might give the physician another level of information. If the patient starts to experience difficulty with bright lights or sounds while doing the maneuvers, for example, that might indicate that there is a migraine headache component to the patient's condition. This finding might also establish the neck as a source of symptoms, as neck injury and migraine are often associated with each other. Having the patient track moving objects with the eyes can help uncover dysfunction of the visual system. Complex balance tasks can get at problems with the vestibular system. These are just a few examples to help you get the point.

While such dynamic physical evaluations can uncover a lot, they also can get pretty complicated. They're necessary, however, if the physician is to get the best possible picture of whether or not PCS is the reason for the patient's symptoms and, if so, what the best approach to improvement will be.

THE UNPLUGGED SYNDROME AND OTHER CONTRIBUTORS TO PCS

Once PCS is identified as the likely cause of an athlete's difficulties, the next step is to use the neurological history and examination to identify all of the contributing factors. Remember, PCS is a collection of symptoms that can come from many potential causes. Now is the time to identify which causes pertain to the current case. Concussion, some of its effects (like poor sleep), and sometimes elements of its management (like over-resting or avoiding social contact) all have a way of adding fuel to any number of preexisting conditions. I have yet to meet a patient whose PCS symptoms had a single generating factor. There has always been some combination of things.

By far, the most common cause of PCS symptoms is what I refer to as the *unplugged syndrome*. This is the longer-term version of the over-resting phenomenon discussed in Chapter 4. As described there, any time a person greatly reduces his physical and cognitive activity, there can be unintended negative effects.

Imagine I told you right now to put this book down (of course I would never really do that!) and go lie down on the couch to rest. Imagine I also told you to avoid any physical activity other than those necessary to sustain life, like eating, drinking, and bathroom breaks, as well as to avoid any mental task, such as reading, texting, using a computer, or watching a movie. I don't want you to go to work or school, and you can't socialize.

Does that sound peaceful? Possibly, given our hectic lives.

Now try staying in that "unplugged" state for four weeks. How do you think you would feel?

Most people would feel lousy, some more than others. Asking an active person such as a student athlete to do this is even worse, and more likely to cause symptoms of fatigue, sleep disturbance, or depression. In this way, the unplugged syndrome becomes the fuel for any other causes of PCS symptoms that are present.

To start figuring out the underlying causes of a patient's PCS (which quite often involves the unplugged syndrome), I make a list of all the factors present, such as sleep, depression, anxiety, and headache. I consider the history and examination further to determine which one of these factors is most likely to be at the core of the syndrome. This is usually not too difficult to determine. It might be a problem that has been there for years, before any concussion, and that has been causing problems by itself. It might be the thing the patient is the most worried about or that's causing the highest level of overall grief. Or it might be combination of these factors.

Once I identify this "mothership" problem I never take my eye off of it. If that central symptom isn't eventually addressed, the patient won't fully recover. The problem is, it's usually not the easiest one of the bunch to treat, and to get the ball rolling it's important to realize some progress.

The next thing I do, therefore, is to identify those factors that can likely be addressed with simple interventions. When you have multiple things at play, all interacting to make one another worse, you need to start somewhere. Once you've achieved one bit of improvement, you can move to another intervention, and then another, and then hopefully you'll have all of the problems moving toward resolution at once.

As you can see, treating PCS can be very complicated. The physician needs to keep an eye on the big picture while attending to all of the smaller things. Sometimes I imagine myself in these situations as a juggler trying to cross a bridge while not dropping anything. I have to attend to each problem to keep them coordinated at the same time, so that I can help the patient as a whole move toward the goal of recovery.

UNTANGLING A KNOT
OF SYMPTOMS

To see how these principles play out in practice, let's return to the story of Anna, the high school soccer player, from the start of this chapter.

Three months after her initial injury, Anna is still symptomatic. Having carefully fleshed out her history, I now suspect that her concussion is more than likely over and she is now suffering from PCS. I have identified that she is clearly fatigued and is having some problems with headache (likely migraine), sleep, and cognition. She also appears to be depressed.

In taking Anna's neurological history, I uncovered a family history of migraine as well as some problems she had with headache at age 13. Combining these findings with the consistency with which she has experienced problems with headache and light sensitivity, I postulate that her underlying, "mothership" problem is migraine headache. Her headaches are being fueled by poor sleep and her depressed mood.

Her sleep difficulties, while still a major problem, are likely a secondary issue brought on by lack of activity and her depressed mood.

Her mood has become a problem because she isn't sleeping, lacks social and cognitive engagement, hasn't been working out, and is emotionally tired from her headaches.

Her cognitive complaints are due to her poor sleep, mood, and headaches.

Her lack of activity feeds each of these and the greater whole—her PCS.

I direct Anna to start an exercise program defined by how she performed in the clinic. She will start slow, simply burning some calories with 20–30 minutes of mild exertion on a stationary bike. She's given clear instructions on how to proceed with increasing her activity.

Once Anna embarks on her exercise program, her mood slowly and consistently begins to turn around as she starts to see some improvement in her overall condition. The uptick is especially noticeable as she increases her physical exertion. Her sleep takes longer to improve, but it eventually does once she's able to tolerate a full day of school without feeling worse.

After a little while, it takes more noise and brighter lights to make her head hurt. For the first time in a month, she has periods of time without head pain.

Almost four months after her initial injury, Anna starts to show recovery from her symptoms. The real fuel to her improvement appears to have been two weeks of consistent sleep.

Through all of this, I consider the different elements of her overall recovery. Melatonin may have helped her sleep. A migraine prevention medication, while lessening her headaches, also may have helped her sleep. Anna also uses over-the-counter anti-inflammatory medications to help with headache. With these interventions, she pulls through her PCS rather easily. Overall, the key to her recovery was early identification and a comprehensive approach to her symptoms and their treatment.

Anna is only one case, of course. The next patient coming through the clinic presents a different set of problems, the most significant being vertigo and balance difficulties (which have been around for eight months!). This patient requires a different solution. That's the nature of PCS. While it's impossible to develop one precise protocol to address all patients, the approach should always be the same: Create an exhaustive list of all possible contributing factors and determine the path forward by taking all of these factors into consideration.

THE FUTURE OF
POST-CONCUSSION SYNDROME

The percentage of people who go on to have PCS after a concussion appears to be increasing. I don't know of any published data supporting this observation, but it does seem to be the case when I look at the patients in our clinic, who represent athletes of all ages and abilities, and when I talk to my colleagues around the country.

If PCS diagnoses really are becoming more common, it might have something to do with heightened awareness. However, it might also reflect more conservative concussion management that inadvertently makes athletes susceptible to PCS by keeping them out of play longer. While I wouldn't ever want to imply that we shouldn't err on the side of being conservative when it comes to concussion, we do need to understand the consequences of our approach.

Moving forward, I think we can do a better job of managing patients with concussion by applying solid neurological principles and producing comprehensive evaluation and management plans. Patients who present with symptoms several weeks after a concussion deserve the best possible care, not the easiest possible care. They deserve to have their lives back, to keep their sense of identity, and to preserve their sense of purpose. Ultimately, I am optimistic that as the medical field becomes more knowledgeable, as the science continues to move forward, and as our approach becomes more refined, PCS will be treated more effectively.

SECOND-IMPACT SYNDROME

From PCS, we now turn to another potential consequence of concussion. You may have heard the term *second-impact syndrome*. It describes a potentially dangerous result of brain trauma, based on the concept that when a brain is in a concussed state, it may be vulnerable to additional and potentially catastrophic injury if exposed to another biomechanical force—a "second hit." The idea is that the second hit causes the already concussed brain to undergo a series of life-threatening changes. In these situations, the brain can swell so much that some brain tissue dies because there isn't enough space in the skull.

Second-impact syndrome was the main driving force behind the introduction of state laws regarding concussion in sports. As discussed in Chapter 3, all 50 states now have some form of concussion legislation designed to protect minors.

Second-impact syndrome is a very serious injury. However, much like other aspects of brain injury, it is often misunderstood and oversimplified.

For example, other injuries can be mistaken for second-impact syndrome. Many sports and recreational activities involve physical risks, and some have very specific risks for brain injury. Sports like football will result in players' taking hits that can produce brain injury. Wrestling, ice hockey, and soccer at any level will too. Throw in recreational activities such as biking, skiing, and snowboarding—all come with similar risks. In reality, the risk of brain injury is around us every single day, whether we play sports or not.

Sometimes these activities produce brain injuries that are more than concussion. They may result in bleeding or significant swelling of the brain. It is entirely possible for these types of injuries to occur without the brain's already being in a concussed state. In these cases it may be tempting to label an injury as second-impact syndrome just because it is very bad. Doing so, however, is inappropriate. While the injury might be an example of second-impact syndrome, it also might have been essentially a one-hit injury. As with most things we've talked about so far, the key to proper diagnosis is to not make assumptions and to take a critical look at the patient's history.

As you might imagine, there is some debate about how common second-impact syndrome really is. Fewer than 20 true, confirmed cases of second-impact syndrome are thought to have been presented in the published, peer-reviewed medical literature. That being said, some people believe that second-impact syndrome is much more common than the low number of verified cases indicates, and they attribute the discrepancy to a lack of awareness of the syndrome.

Regardless of the true numbers, second-impact syndrome should be considered one more important reason why no person who is suspected of having a concussion should be allowed to continue an activity with brain trauma risk, and why no one with a diagnosed concussion should be allowed to return to participating in a contact sport until the medical personnel overseeing his or her care are as certain as possible that the concussion is over.

In the end, my best advice to any athlete with a suspected concussion or possible PCS, or to the parent of such an athlete, is simple. Find a physician with experience taking care of neurological disorders—preferably one with experience in the particular issue of brain trauma in athletes. Have that doctor not only help you through the injury but also consider your overall brain health. Establish an ongoing relationship with that doctor. One thing I feel is critically important, especially for athletes who play a contact or collision sport, is to have an annual evaluation of your brain health. Be proactive and be prepared. There are a lot of benefits from playing sports, and we want you playing them as long as you can.

Six

Concussion, Sports, Depression, and Suicide

Former NFL quarterback Eric Hipple played high school football decades before our high school star from Chapter I, Spencer Helgren, stepped onto the field. Hipple's football talent turned into his career, while Spencer now fondly looks back on his high school playing days as he enjoys college. Still, Hipple readily identifies with today's youth players. He understands their mindset of playing through pain. Trying to act like everything is fine even when it is clearly not is a struggle endured by all driven athletes, no matter the level of play, their age, or their gender.

Hipple, now in his 50s and a good distance away from his football-playing days, has the mature perspective to realize that when he was in high school, he was trying to live up a self-created ideal, one where he, as the star quarterback, couldn't ever be injured. He wouldn't admit to injury, and he kept going no matter what happened. He enjoyed the pressure. He was the most important player on his team, serving as the focal point of the game and the fans. That bright spotlight, which could be problematic for some people, was Hipple's source of self-confidence. It carried a potent form of social status, a type of calling card Hipple felt he could build his fragile, evolving teen identity around. He felt invincible and powerful on the field, using the rush of playing football and being a blue-chip, college-bound quarterback in California to mask what was happening to him off the field.

Hipple, like many teens and preteens, was actually dealing with beginnings of a serious battle with depression. He traces his first signs of depression back to junior high, where he felt moments of anxiety and, sometimes, overpowering periods of sadness and self-doubt while trying to navigate social, home, and classroom situations. He says he never felt like anything he did was good enough and lived in fear of judgment from peers, family, and teachers. He worried they would discover he was not strong, smart, or worthy of respect.

But football was different. It became his haven, a place where depression didn't seem to touch him. Playing sports, and excelling at them—thanks to his talent as a strong and intuitive athlete—was a way to hide from what was going on in other parts of his life. Being an athlete also gave him purpose and a set schedule of tasks. Nobody would ever think the star quarterback could be anything but happy all the time.

Hipple did have concussions, both from playing football and from a car crash, further complicating his struggles with untreated depression and growing thoughts of suicide. Depression followed him throughout his career regardless of whether or not he was injured—but it certainly got worse in times of injury. His depression became even more acute when he was told he would no longer be an NFL quarterback. There was no more hiding on a football field, no creation of an alternate reality away from depression. He had suffered symptoms away from the game, during his game-playing years, and after he was done playing the game that he loved.

Hipple finally got help, and he has become an outspoken advocate for others who have depression—especially athletes and youth. His willingness to speak out about being a star athlete living with depression serves as a powerful lesson for all of us.

"The macho idea that guys who are athletes can't be depressed [and] overcome whatever comes their way because they are tough is really dumb and we need to change that discussion," Hipple says. "I know of a lot of guys who are in same spot where I used to be, and being a star in the NFL or whatever you are, even as a young athlete, is not going to mean everything is OK. We need to be able to say, as athletes, as people, that 'I need help.' It took a long time for me to get there."

"Depression," like "concussion," is a term that gets thrown around a lot in the world of sports. As a topic, it's often presented side by side with suicide as an inevitable outcome of playing contact sports. But the relationships between concussion, depression, and suicide are more complex than is typically acknowledged on the news or around the cyber–water coolers of the Internet.

There are important differences between *depression* as a feeling or symptom, being *clinically depressed*, and having a diagnosis of *depressive disorder*. We often hear commentators on the news use those terms interchangeably and without much regard for the nuances of their meanings. If we truly want to understand how sports, depression, and suicide might be related, it's critical to know what those words mean, how they are abused, and how to use them, and in what contexts, to best get accurate messages across. Let's explore them, starting with some simple definitions and examples.

DEPRESSION WITH A LITTLE "d"

Standing on its own, the term *depression* simply means what it sounds like: feeling depressed or sad, or having a depressed mood. You can be naturally depressed for a lot of reasons without there being any underlying abnormal condition. When your youngest child moves away from home, you're likely to feel some degree of sadness. Reacting to the death of a loved one is another form. Depression is a very normal feeling, one that occurs in all of us at times. If we have an expected amount of sadness in reaction to an emotional circumstance, that condition should not be considered in any way abnormal, even given the wide range of what a "normal" amount of sadness can be within the human population.

Individuals who have a concussion will often describe feeling sad or having a depressed mood. This is one of the common symptoms that physicians and athletic trainers look for when evaluating a concussed or potentially concussed athlete. This brings up yet another tricky aspect of concussion care: The sadness or depressed mood could be coming from either or both of two separate mechanisms.

First, the injury itself could be disrupting the brain networks that are responsible for the athlete's mood, directly causing the feeling of sadness. Second, the athlete may be feeling sad about his or her situation. Simply being injured is an extremely common reason to feel sad or depressed. We see this not only in athletes but in anybody with a significant injury that is causing pain or dysfunction or making the person miss school, sports, work, or social activities. The important thing to remember about this cause of sadness is that is not abnormal. It is a natural reaction to a bad situation. With this in mind, I always ask my concussed patients who are experiencing sadness or a depressed mood how they have reacted emotionally in previous times of injury.

Whether caused organically by the injury or as an emotional reaction, the depression or sadness experienced with a concussion is very real and should be taken seriously. It is common enough that all people with a concussion, no matter their age or gender, should be asked about it. I'll talk more about treating depression a little bit later in this chapter.

CLINICAL DEPRESSION

Let's compare this first situation with clinical depression. It's quite important to know the difference between the two and to be able to figure out which one is in play in a concussed patient. While depression is most accurately considered a normal human response to a situation, clinical depression consists of sadness or depressed mood that occurs without provocation or is out of proportion in severity or duration to any potentially depression-causing situation currently present. Clinical depression should be considered an abnormal state of emotional control. Although not as common as simply experiencing the feeling of being depressed, clinical depression is quite common throughout many stages of life.

A potentially helpful way to look at clinical depression is to consider it as a condition of a person's mood that began after some event and then took on a life of its own. It is as if the triggering event opened a cage, letting the depressed mood free to act on its own accord. Just like the symptom of depression, common life events, such as divorce, retirement, or other personal loss, can lead to clinical depression. Concussion can too. The depression we discussed in Chapter 5 as a common component of post-concussion syndrome is a form of clinical depression.

MAJOR DEPRESSIVE DISORDER

When somebody has a problem with mood regulation that meets a very particular medical definition, they are given a very specific diagnosis: major depressive disorder (MDD). This diagnosis is specific for good reason: Clinically, we need to be able to distinguish patients with MDD from those who have clinical depression or are simply depressed as a normal reaction. Patients with MDD typically require a comprehensive psychiatric approach and well-tailored therapy. The definition of MDD used by medical professionals comes from the American Psychiatric Association's *Diagnostic and Statistical Manual of Mental Disorders*. Key criteria for an MDD diagnosis include experiencing a depressed mood for more than two weeks that represents a notable change from the person's baseline mood and that impairs social, occupational, or academic function while producing significant outward effects such as irritability, fatigue, loss of energy, or weight change. Major depressive disorder can be a chronic or recurrent problem that requires continuity of medical care.

When we hear in news reports or quick-take Tweets that concussions or playing contact sports leads to depression, it's important to think critically about what point the person using the term is trying to make. Is the word being used to describe the feeling of sadness that often comes with being concussed?

Maybe it refers to the clinical depression that often sets in after an athlete is forced to retire from sports? More and more, however, you'll notice that conversations referring to "depression" are actually talking about the diagnosis of MDD.

Of course, to make matters even more complicated, it's absolutely possible for someone to be suffering from all three kinds of depression. Individuals with MDD can certainly experience increased sadness in response to circumstances or have an episode of clinical depression.

KEEPING IT ALL STRAIGHT

As you might guess, it can be very confusing for patients, families, and medical care providers when all three kinds of depression are present at the same time.

Let's use the example of Zach, an athlete in his early teens who has a preexisting MDD diagnosis, or maybe has the disorder but has yet to be diagnosed. Zach is doing OK in the face of his depression, but not great. However, he and his family both note that Zach's mood has definitely been better since he started playing organized sports. This change shouldn't be a surprise, as physical activity is a well-studied and widely accepted moderator of depressed mood. In addition, being part of team or competing in a solo sport can create a positive sense of self and accomplishment. So Zach's sports activity is a major boost to his mood in several ways.

Still, our teen athlete has MDD. Zach took medication for depression in the past but has stopped since beginning regular and frequent psychotherapy. His grades are good enough, and he has a social life, if not exactly a healthy or stable one.

Now imagine Zach gets concussed during a practice. It happens in a routine play, but there is contact to the head. He says something about the event to his head coach, who in turn lets Zach's parents know that he has a possible concussion. In addition to experiencing headache and sleep difficulty, Zach's mood changes and worsens, so much so that he does not want to leave the house.

Further, it turns out this isn't Zach's first concussion—it's his third. The previous two also happened while he was playing sports, one over two years ago and the first one four years ago. As happened with those previous injuries, he recovers significantly over roughly two weeks. With this injury, however, he has yet to shake his nagging sadness. In every other way, Zach has recovered, and he is nearly back to his pre-injury state academically and socially. He hasn't been given clearance to return to his sport yet. Actually, he's been told not to do any physical activity other than what's necessary for routine daily living.

Our young athlete's parents then seek the advice of a clinician who can help them decide if it's safe for him to return to play. Well-intentioned friends have already told them that because this is his third concussion, retirement is Zach's best option. Looking for evidence to support a recommendation, the clinician cites a common belief, "The more concussions you have, the more depression you have." He recommends retirement.

So Zach now prepares for a life after sport. He looks for a replacement activity, something that can provide the same sense of identity that he got from playing a sport and being part of a team, but he finds none. Zach tries to stay physically active, but he struggles to find a reason and purpose. His mood worsens, and his motivation becomes nonexistent. Finding the energy and focus to work on academics becomes more difficult. Zach's grades begin to suffer, further eroding an already delicate self-image. A clinical depression sets in, one that is deep and difficult to treat. As time goes on and his depressive symptoms continue to worsen, Zach's parents fear that his retirement from sports came too late. They conclude, based on both popular thought and the medical recommendation their son received, that his history of concussion and playing sports is the cause of his current situation. In other words, the last concussion was the final straw.

Zach feels like he is broken beyond repair, with hope fading for a normal life. It's a nightmare scenario for any parent or youth athlete.

But what actually led Zach to this point? Was it his history of concussions? Or if not the concussions themselves, maybe the other, "smaller" hits along the way made things worse? Currently, there's no way to test individuals for the latter effect, but there is enough data to suggest that both concussions and repetitive hits may make depression worse. This is not clear-cut, however, and the possibility should be considered on a case-by-case basis.

Stepping back, it's important to note that the oft-cited belief that a history of concussion leads to depression, as assumed in the nightmare scenario, has scarce scientific evidence to support it. The relationship between a history of concussion and the risk of developing depression has been explored mainly through a series of self-reported, retrospective surveys that sometimes have asked athletes to recall diagnoses they were given decades before. Individuals are more likely to receive a concussion diagnosis if they already have a history of concussion, so this becomes a chicken-and-egg problem. Also, because the medical history patients provide is always colored by what they are experiencing emotionally, depression may bias how people recall their past injuries.

At the same time, there is little doubt that retiring from sports at any age can have profound negative effects on a person's psychology. Zach's problems with depression stemmed primarily from his removal from sports and not from injuries he sustained while playing it. This became apparent after he underwent a comprehensive neurological evaluation whose results led to a multifaceted rehabilitation process. Zach was given a very specific tailored rehab regimen in addition to medications to help with his depression. Gradually he began to feel better, and after several weeks Zach did return to his sport. At this point, his mood had improved to his pre-concussion baseline.

This is not to say that anybody should continue with a sport that is unsafe just to avoid the depression that comes with no longer playing it. Rather, it's necessary to consider both sides of the equation and strive to understand all of the risks that might lead to depression. It's also necessary to be aware of which claims or assumptions represent hype or misunderstandings. Only then can one arrive at a truly informed judgment about retiring from a sport.

SUICIDE AND SPORTS

Unfortunately, suicide is a part of the human experience. And it is sadly an all-too-common one. According to the Centers for Disease Control and Prevention (CDC),[1] 41,149 people took their own lives in the United States in 2013, more than the number of deaths resulting from car accidents (32,719, according to the National Highway Traffic Safety Administration[2]). According to a 2011 CDC report, suicide is the third leading cause of death for children in the 10- to 14-year-old age group, and the second leading cause for those 15–34 years old.[3]

Sports usually reflect what's going on in society, and of course suicide touches athletes as well as the general public. There's nothing magical about being a well-known athlete that insulates you from the things that can lead to suicide. That said, when a member of our society who is known for physical abilities, mental toughness, and a competitive edge takes his or her own life, it somehow feels different and more shocking. There's a sense of disbelief as we try to reconcile this outcome with what we knew, or assumed we knew, about the person. Understanding and accepting any suicide is difficult, but it seems even more so when it involves one of our sports heroes. However, these people are not invincible, unlike the superhero image created by our society.

Dave Duerson was a very successful professional football player. He played safety for the Chicago Bears, New York Giants, and Phoenix Cardinals during a career that spanned the years 1983 to 1993. He died on February 17, 2011, at the age of 50, after shooting himself fatally in the chest. Before doing so, he left a note for his family asking that his brain be donated to a research group known to be looking into the link between chronic traumatic encephalopathy (CTE) and a lifetime of playing contact sports. His brain was examined, and it was indeed found to have changes that the researchers concluded were from his years in football. The narrative was powerful, stunning, and reported repeatedly: Duerson's sports career had led to brain damage, which then caused him to take his own life.

The message from Duerson's case started a steady drumbeat: Football was responsible for taking the lives of its star players.

Junior Seau had an even longer NFL career than Duerson, starring for 19 years as a linebacker known for his physical play. He was widely known as an exceptional player and teammate and earned 12 trips to the Pro Bowl. Seau was charismatic, almost larger than life—on and off the field. But he came to the same fate as Duerson, taking his own life at the age of 43 on May 2, 2012. Perhaps primed by the earlier death of Duerson, Seau's story was discussed even more widely, throughout every corner of our society and media, becoming an integral part of the national conversation on concussions in sports. His brain was examined by a different group of researchers from the ones who had autopsied Duerson's, but the pathologists reached the same conclusion: Playing football had led to changes in Seau's brain. They couldn't comment on whether or not those changes led to his suicide, because the science doesn't exist to do that. The narrative, however, was already established and clear to the world: Playing football had damaged another star player in a way that caused him to take his own life.

Owen Thomas never reached the elite level of professional football. He was a collegiate player when he took his own life on April 26, 2010, at the age of 21. His teammates at the University of Pennsylvania had just voted him captain for the upcoming season. Thomas's brain was examined after death and found to have the same types of changes as Duerson's and Seau's—although to a much lesser degree. Despite caution from many in the medical world about reaching unsubstantiated conclusions, his case was widely publicized as another example where football led to suicide.

Each of these cases is heartbreaking, a wrenching loss of a person who leaves behind grieving family members, friends, and teammates. Each makes us pause and wonder what led these individuals to such a dark place. It's natural to want to explain suicide, to look for a cause. The need to find the "why" is usually especially acute for the survivors, who often are dealing with grief, hurt, and confusion and who may harbor significant feelings of guilt. Fans as well want to understand why a beloved, dynamic athlete, even a retired one, would end her or his life.

There is a tremendous amount of research on the causes and conditions that lead to suicide attempts. One thing is clear from this research: There isn't a simple explanation for why people take their own lives. Rather, it is often the case that many factors come together at once.

SUICIDE CONTAGION

We know that suicide is all too common. As a public health issue, it also has been shown to be influenced by how openly it's talked about in the public and media. Simply put, news about one individual's suicide can lead others to commit suicide. In one famous instance of such "suicide contagion," the suicide rate in the United States in 1962 jumped by 12 percent over a period of three months as compared with the year before. The explanation? While it is difficult to prove a causal link, the increase occurred in the months that followed the death by suicide of Marilyn Monroe.

In the summer of 2015, former NFL star quarterback Eric Kramer tried to take his own life. He was found in time by paramedics and survived the suicide attempt. Chatter immediately sprung up in social media about the shocking news, with the focus turning to the by-now-established equation that football = concussions = CTE = suicide. Instead of the outright horror that stemmed from Seau's and Duerson's deaths, there was more of an attitude of acceptance, bordering on indifference, that suicide was a predicable outcome for football players. Kramer played football, so it "made sense" that he would attempt suicide.

That concept is so wrong, on so many levels.

The medical community has long realized that suicide rates can be affected by messaging. The effect is even more compelling when that messaging is based on assumptions and oversimplifications. In 1994, the Centers for Disease Control and Prevention released a report entitled *Suicide Contagion and the Reporting of Suicide*.[4] The report represented not only the judgment of a multidisciplinary panel of suicide experts but also the findings from a careful review of published medical literature. The report contained the following recommendations for preventing suicide contagion:

Do NOT:

1. Present simplistic explanations for suicide
2. Engage in repetitive, ongoing, or excessive reporting of suicide in the news

3. Provide sensational coverage of suicide
4. Report "how-to" descriptions of suicide
5. Present suicide as a tool for accomplishing certain ends
6. Glorify suicide or persons who commit suicide
7. Focus on the suicide completer's positive characteristics.

Each of these acts was felt to increase the chances that somebody who is at risk of committing suicide will do so. This would naturally drive up the suicide rate in the population.

As can be seen from multiple examples in the media, like that of Kramer, and even in the medical community, a lot of people are not following this advice when talking about suicide in athletes. Unlike the isolated case of a single Hollywood icon taken from us in the prime of her career, professional athletes are perceived to be linked together as a group. In other words, iconic Monroe's headline-dominating death is nothing compared with the constant messaging and reporting that occur each time a professional athlete commits suicide.

SUICIDE RATES IN NATIONAL FOOTBALL LEAGUE PLAYERS

There may be some evidence of suicide contagion among football players. In 2012 researchers from the National Institute for Occupational Safety and Health (NIOSH) published a study that looked at the relationship between certain health conditions and cardiac causes of death in NFL players who had played for at least five years between 1959 and 1988. Though the study focused on heart disease, the NIOSH researchers also reported the number of suicides that had occurred in these 3,439 former NFL players. The data collection period ended in 2007. At that time, this group of ex-football players had a suicide rate that was less than half that for a general population sample that matched the players in age and gender.[5]

Surprising?

Yes—especially when we take a look at what has happened in the population of former NFL players since 2008.

From the NIOSH study, we know that between 1979 and 2007 there were 9 suicides among former NFL players, or 0.19 per year. Between 2008 and the writing of this book in 2015, there have been 11, or 1.6 per year.

That's more than an eightfold increase in the suicide rate.

What's the difference between these two time periods? What changed around 2008? One obvious answer is the increased focus on athletes' suicides in the media, pop culture, and Hollywood. Another contributor might be changes in the financial reimbursement that players receive and the societal adjustment they undergo on retiring. When players leave football today, they typically have a larger gap than older players did between the money they made while playing and what they make after leaving the game, and they experience a greater loss of fame. Going back to "normal life" can be jarring for these former athletes. They are left searching for meaning for their life off the field.

THE BIGGER PICTURE

I told the above stories about the suicides of football players, two professional and one collegiate, and discussed the statistics for former NFL players to illustrate a point. Suicide is not a problem only among football players. Not at all. Football players are, however, the subject of the loudest and most frequently repeated narrative about suicide in athletes. Therefore this is also the story that my patients and their parents hear most often, the one they carry around in their minds every day, and the one that brings them to my clinic.

Over the past five or six years, I have witnessed a clear increase in concerns about suicide in my patients, with significant focus from athletes who have been diagnosed with concussion. These fears are often cited as a reason to avoid sports altogether, not just the contact variety.

Depression is a condition, one with many causes. Suicide is, unfortunately, an endpoint, also with many causes. To oversimplify and misrepresent the complexity of these two phenomena is not only inaccurate but frankly quite dangerous. With today's nonstop barrage of social media and 24-hour news cycles, how many young athletes, adult athletes, and former athletes do you think hear about the purported chain that links sports, depression, and suicide every day? How many of those individuals are depressed? Depression is estimated to effect at least 1 in 10 of all Americans. That's nearly 32 million people.

I only ask that as much as we care about the effects of brain trauma on depression and suicide, we also care about the words we use and the way we use them when we talk about those effects. How we approach this issue can absolutely make a difference. The message matters.

TREATING DEPRESSION IN ATHLETES

Understanding the root cause of someone's depression is essential to treating it effectively. Depression is real, and depression is treatable. And making sure that depressed people receive treatment should be a goal for all of us.

It's also important to keep in mind that depression can affect any athlete, any person, at any time. So the annual pre-participation physical or medical checkup is also a great time to look into the possible presence of a mood issue like depression.

As noted above, the period following a concussion is another good time to keep an eye out for symptoms of depression. Typically, the depression that results from the concussion itself doesn't need to be treated with medication or any type of direct intervention, because like the other symptoms of concussion it is usually short-lived.

In some cases, however, a clinical depression sets in that outlives the direct effects of the injury itself. It then becomes essential to have the patient evaluated by a medical professional trained in dealing with mood disorders. Medications may be indicated or not, depending on the case. Counseling, cognitive therapy, or other forms of psychotherapy may be helpful. Having an open mind about potential factors and treatment is key for patient improvement. In this situation, inactivity is the enemy. Social and physical engagement is essential.

Sometimes a concussion can uncover a more serious MDD, which will likely require a longer period of treatment. Individuals who fit this description must be evaluated comprehensively.

In all three of these scenarios, there will be times when certain activities, such as contact sports, should be avoided and times when they may be an essential component of recovery.

A LIFE REGAINED

Ben Gur-Arie was a successful freshman quarterback at Ann Arbor Huron High School. He was well liked by his peers, enjoyed school, and got good grades. He seemed to be on a good path. However, after the football season ended during his first year of high school, he found himself hanging more often with the "wrong crowd." Looking for something to take the place of football, he discovered alcohol, drugs, and some new friends to go with his new habits. Looking back now, Ben and his parents realize he was likely self-treating an underlying problem with depression.

As the school year went on, his grades suffered. By the end of his freshman year, Ben found himself academically ineligible to play sports. His destructive behaviors continued through the summer and into his sophomore year, and he now was without sports as an outlet. One night he swiped vodka from his parents' liquor cabinet, poured it into water bottle to hide the clear liquid, and took the family car to meet with friends. He was drinking heavily and admits he doesn't clearly remember much of that fateful night.

Ben drove recklessly, and instead of turning left or right when the street dead-ended at a stop sign, he continued straight ahead—too fast. He plowed the family car into a sign, the violence of the crash driving the metal signpost through the windshield. Ben's skull was impaled by the metal. He was seriously injured and required a long stay in the intensive care unit. It took multiple surgeries to save his life and restore his skull and facial bone structure.

Ben had a long road to recovery from what turned out to be a significant brain injury. He had to relearn simple tasks. Ben spent several weeks in the hospital and many more in outpatient rehabilitation.

But he did recover function and regained his health well enough to return to school full-time. He was clearly scarred, both physically and emotionally. He had problems with sleep, concentration, and memory, all thought to be clear effects of his traumatic brain injury. In spite of all of this, Ben was able to keep up academically. He was not, however, playing football.

During December of his junior year, the football coach approached Ben in the cafeteria during lunch with a simple question: "Are you ready?"

Up until that point, Ben hadn't considered playing football again. It didn't seem to be a possibility, given all he had been through in his recovery. And obviously, with his complex injuries there was a lot to consider. I was asked to see him, to address his medical issues and determine whether it would be safe for him to play again. I performed a detailed medical evaluation to help decide that question.

As amazing as it seems, Ben did return to football the next summer. In his first game as the starting quarterback, he led his team to an overtime victory. More important by far were the unintended consequences of his return. His mood improved, as did his sleep. With those changes came an improvement in overall energy, attention, and memory. In essence, all of things he experienced after his accident that had been attributed to brain injury were not from the accident at all. They arose directly from the loss he felt from not playing football.

REFERENCES

1. Xu JQ, Murphy SL, Kochanek KD, Bastian BA. *Deaths: Final Data for 2013.* Hyattsville, MD: National Center for Health Statistics; 2016. National Vital Statistics Reports 64, no. 2. http://www.cdc.gov/nchs/data/nvsr/nvsr64/nvsr64_02.pdf.
2. *2013 Motor Vehicle Crashes: Overview.* Washington, DC: National Highway Traffic Safety Administration, National Center for Statistics and Analysis; December 2014. Traffic Safety Facts Research Note. Report no. DOT HS 812 101. http://www-nrd.nhtsa.dot.gov/Pubs/812101.pdf.
3. *Suicide: Facts at a Glance 2015.* Atlanta, GA: Centers for Disease Control and Prevention, National Center for Injury Prevention and Control, Division of Violence Prevention. http://www.cdc.gov/violenceprevention/pdf/suicide-datasheet-a.pdf.
4. O'Carroll PW, Potter LB, Aronowitz E, et al. Suicide contagion and the reporting of suicide: recommendations from a national workshop. *MMWR Recommendations and Reports* April 22, 1994;43(RR-6):9–18. http://www.cdc.gov/mmwr/preview/mmwr html/00031539.htm.
5. Lehman E. Brain injury in the NFL. September 6, 2012. http://blogs.cdc.gov/niosh-science-blog/2012/09/06/nfl-brain-injury/.

SEVEN

How Athletes Can Help Themselves

It's fascinating to consider the psyche of a highly successful athlete. No matter the age—10 years old, 25, or the 45-year-old weekend warrior—many such individuals seem to possess certain traits, beyond natural talent and physical attributes, that separate them from the average athlete. Some of these traits are likely innate, while others are created and honed through years of practice and play.

Mental toughness, sharp focus, the ability to play through pain, and a pronounced willingness to take risks, even when they're not logical or obvious choices, set the truly special athletes apart from their peers. Former high school football player Spencer Helgren, profiled in Chapter 1, admits he was willing to try to play through a possible concussion. Quitting was an option he would never consider. Former high school, now varsity college cheerleader Kristin Johnson quashed her fears about safety and levels of preparation during tough flying stunts to meet her own standards of being a good teammate and keeping the respect of her peers. And some of the superstars who were able to make their childhood sports passions into their adult jobs, like two-time Olympic gold medalist and World Cup–winning soccer player Kate (née Sobrero) Markgraf and pioneering X Games snowboarder Ellery Hollingsworth, acknowledge that they played through pain and injury.

Markgraf and Hollingsworth, both now retired from their super-elite professional sports careers, also admit their passion led to multiple concussions. Often athletes do not want to accept they can get hurt, because it might pierce the thick cloak of confidence they need to wear to be successful. Being stronger, tougher, and braver is always the name of the game. Admitting a weakness, even it is merely admitting to being a human being who can get hurt, is not in their lexicon. Coaches preach toughness and bravado, parents can reinforce the message, and peer pressure among teammates locks in the concept. Being hurt or being fearful of being hurt could make an athlete more risk adverse or tentative. Being hesitant means not taking that last-second shot, not cutting that slalom gate a little closer, not laying your body out for the critical tackle.

Hollingsworth, Markgraf, Johnson, Helgren, and Eric Hipple from Chapter 6 come from different backgrounds, generations, and sports, but nowadays they have the same message for youth athletes, from Pee Wee football players to those of Olympic caliber, and for their parents and coaches: If you even think you might be injured, say something to somebody. Please. Athletes are not indestructible, they can get concussed, and they need to be honest when they are hurt.

"I never wanted to admit I was hurt, not to my mom, not to my coaches, really, to nobody," Helgren says. "When I had my first concussion in a game, all I wanted to do was keep playing. I went back in, got hit again, and I still wanted to keep playing. You get told to play through pain, to go for it. They asked me how I was, and I told them I was fine, even though I wasn't.

"I believed I should keep playing because I didn't want to let my team down. But I didn't make the right decisions, because staying in the game wasn't smart for my health."

In my experience as a clinician, it's not unusual for athletes, whether in youth leagues or professionals, to work through a thought process denying the possibility or evidence of injury. They will "talk themselves out of" having a concussion or any other type of injury, trying to hide symptoms because they are scared and fear negative reactions should their coaches, teammates, or parents find out they're hurt. They often think they are skilled enough at controlling their bodies and minds to hide something like being dazed or dizzy on the field. We know that the concussed brain frequently does not allow the athlete to make logical choices.

But none of this deception of themselves or others is worth the potential lifetime consequences for their brain of ignoring injury. If athletes are hurt, if they do not feel right, if they know in their gut that something is wrong, they should feel empowered to say something. Telling their coaches, teammates, or family members what they think those people want to hear doesn't help anybody in the end. Coaches and parents should want their athletes to be strong, healthy, and able to have a great life in—and out of—sports. The attitude of coaches and parents is changing, as we'll discuss in Chapter 8, but often the message to be proactive about concussions can get lost or is willfully ignored.

The challenge is often to get athletes of any age to think the right way about concussion safety.

PUSHING THE BOUNDARIES

Hollingsworth heard that concussions were a big deal more than a few times. Her coaches mentioned it. Her mom, Linherr, made her wear an uncool-looking ski helmet while she zipped down the halfpipe as a child in her native Vermont. (Back then, wearing a helmet while skiing was not fashionable.)

"I was fearless, and being scared or conservative wasn't going to be me," Hollingsworth says. "Getting hurt was just something that happened, you got up and kept going, and concussions were something that happened to other people."

She was laser-focused on becoming a champion snowboarder, which meant daily hard falls, occasionally hitting her head, and sometimes feeling weird. As she progressed in snowboarding, her skills and tricks evolved to riskier levels so that she could compete for gold medals, ultimately aiming for the Olympics and X Games. Hollingsworth's fearlessness helped her become the first female snowboarder to land a "1080": a high-risk, high-strength, and high–body control move that involves spinning through multiple revolutions—sometimes while twisting at the same time—as you fly through the air, launched off the edge of the quarter pipe or halfpipe. Her 1080, which she pulled off in 2009 when she was only 17, was a revolutionary moment in snowboarding that propelled her into one of the biggest names in the sport.

Hollingsworth was the golden girl of snowboarding, with fans loving her for her open and fun personality, her clear talent, her willingness to take risks, and her thrilling runs that blew the crowds away every time she competed.

She now reluctantly remembers a few hard falls during practice, admitting that she purposely tried to forget most of them to master the 1080. She snowboarded hurt. But she couldn't ignore everything around her. The fate-altering snowboarding accidents of close friends, along with her growing awareness of the number of crashes she was regularly sustaining, changed everything for her. Hollingsworth's boyfriend, US snowboarder Kevin Pearce, ended up in a coma with a severe traumatic brain injury from a superpipe crash while training for the 2010 Winter Olympics.[1] Pearce's accident shocked the world of skiing and snowboarding. One minute he was being promoted as one of the possible stars of the Vancouver Olympics; the next he was fighting for his life, and the world was discussing the dangers of superpipe. Thankfully Pearce has since recovered, but he no longer competes.

But the losses were not over. Two years later, on the same superpipe in Park City, Utah, where Pearce had been hurt, Canadian star Sarah Burke, a friendly competitor of Hollingsworth's, sustained a fatal brain injury after crashing violently during a training run on January 19, 2012.[2]

Hollingsworth retired in 2014, at age 22. Her dream of being part of the US Olympic team for the 2014 Winter Games in Sochi, Russia, an Olympics where experts viewed her as a serious medal contender, was taken away because of post-concussive issues and her desire to protect her brain from further damage. She could not compete in Sochi because a month before the Olympics she started sliding into a sequence of migraines, sleep problems, and depression-like symptoms. Her health dramatically changed her priorities.

Hollingsworth has a message to share with today's young athletes who think themselves to be as fearless as she once was.

"You think because you are younger and healthy that nothing can happen," she says. "And when it does happen, you think you just shake it off and keep going.

"Getting older taught me fear, after seeing what happened to my friends pushing the envelope in the sport. You can't do what I was doing if you have fear, because it stops you. I knew I had to make a decision, and I did. I have no regrets."

Hollingsworth has regained her health and has a bright future after sports, thanks to working with her doctors. (Full disclosure: I was one of them.) She has redefined her priorities in sport and life and is now a full-time college honors student majoring in marketing. Retiring from snowboarding, something she has been passionate about since she was six, wasn't easy. She says her sponsors have been understanding about her choice to step away from competition, and she may want to find a way to stay in snowboarding on the business or design side.

Hollingsworth doesn't think she ever deliberately lied to her coaches or parents about possibly being concussed. But she also didn't actively volunteer to talk about the hard crashes she had at practice or during competitions. She says she feels lucky to have received good care from US Skiing and Snowboarding that allowed her to feel confident about safely going back out to compete after a fall.

"I want us to have a more open world where we can talk about being hurt and not be afraid of anything," Hollingsworth says. "I never thought I should admit to being hurt, because that meant I wasn't strong. Or I wouldn't be back competing because somebody would have to check me out. I didn't think I had time for that. I wanted to keep going."

KNOWING YOUR LIMITS

Markgraf reached the highest levels of her sport and became a starting defender on the highly successful and very popular US women's soccer team from 1999 to 2008. She played in 201 international games and earned a reputation for toughness and smarts on the soccer pitch. In many ways, Markgraf, along with teammates such as Mia Hamm, Julie Foudy, and Michelle Akers, put US women's soccer into the mainstream and drove the swell of popularity of soccer that is still growing among the American public.

Like Hollingsworth, Markgraf achieved her elite status by sometimes playing through pain. Playing in the World Cup, the Olympics, and numerous tournaments and "friendlies" put Markgraf up against the best soccer players in the world. The game at that level is played fairly cleanly but still comes with hard collisions when players are going for the ball, elbows while players are jostling for position, and rough falls. Markgraf has paid the price for standing her ground and playing tough defense, suffering seven diagnosed concussions.

Markgraf, who retired from the US national team in 2008 and pro soccer in 2010, admits her competitiveness sometimes got in the way of her better judgment.

"You play in the moment, in the game, and do what you have been training to do, so no, you're not giving a second to think, 'Maybe what I just did is going to result in a concussion,'" Markgraf says. "When you're at something like the Olympics or the World Cup, you take what is happening on the field and move on. You can't let yourself focus on every bump or bruise that you get."

Markgraf is happy that concussion awareness has changed dramatically since she started in the game. She doesn't recall much formal discussion of concussion and neurological awareness during her days starting for the

University of Notre Dame in the mid-1990s—even though she knows players were being concussed in practices or games. The attitude of being tougher than any injury and the lack of understanding that the brain can be injured from soccer were hallmarks of that earlier era.

"There really wasn't any talk about concussions in soccer when I started, like there is now—it just never came up for some reason. Maybe we just didn't know enough back then," Markgraf says. "I still see we need more discussion at all levels, from youth on up to the national team, about it. I still think there is a lot more the athletes need to know and think about."

Markgraf traces most of her concussions to collisions in soccer. She has broken her nose several times, the result of going for the ball against another player or running into an accidental elbow. Once, in 2000, she was knocked out while playing, recovered on the sidelines, and still tried to re-enter the game despite being likely concussed. She also has gone through a three-month bout with post-concussion syndrome (PCS).

Being more aware of concussions and their impact came into play during the last year of Markgraf's professional career. It was 2010, and she was playing for the Chicago Red Stars in the Women's Professional Soccer league. She had taken a blow to the head, nothing on the same scale as previous collisions, but it still led to another concussion. She sat out for few days to recover, but she knew her team needed her back on the pitch. They were stronger if she was playing. And her veteran competitive instincts guided her into wanting to play.

But her heart was telling her something else. She knew she had to be evaluated by a doctor before she could be put back on the active roster.

"I was so relieved when the doctor would not clear me to play," Markgraf recalls. "It took the decision out of my hands, and I knew it was the right decision. I was in no shape to play. But I wasn't going to admit that, I was going to be tough and try to play. I wasn't going to let my team down. But having a good doctor look at everything, and tell me the truth, was critical.

"I think that could be the difference for a lot of athletes, to have the right medical staff advocating for their health and making decisions."

For an athlete, being honest about feeling strange or knowing that you're hurt can be scary. Depending on the athlete's age, it can also be a challenge to state what is wrong. An 11-year-old can articulate how he thinks he may be injured or describe how he is feeling but may choose not to say anything. On the other hand, a 5-year-old may be more honest in her reaction to an injury but not as able to precisely describe what's wrong.

Kristin Johnson spent most of her childhood as a gymnast. She loved the artistic side of the sport, along with the challenge of the acrobatics. She knew the potential for injury existed in gymnastics, usually from accidents on the apparatuses. She decided to channel her gymnastics skills in a different direction when she entered high school in Rochester, Michigan, by going into competitive cheerleading. Johnson's small frame and advanced gymnastics training made her a natural to become a flyer—the cheerleader who is thrown into the air to execute flips, twists, and pikes during competitive routines and during the quick performances during breaks in football and basketball games. Being accidentally dropped or being caught in an awkward fashion was an everyday fear that Johnson learned to negotiate through denial.

"Sometimes you get that feeling that something isn't right, or you are trying some big skill too fast without taking the right steps to practice it," says Johnson, who is now a varsity cheerleader at the University of Michigan and was part of the 2014–16 teams that have won the national competitive cheer title. "I think when you are younger, you swallow those doubts and don't tell anybody that you are scared or unsure about what you are doing. It's like you just go with it and hope it will all turn out OK, like you will figure it all out as you go. Which is stupid. If you have doubts about something, it's probably because something is off."

Johnson says she was lucky to get through gymnastics and high school cheer without any significant injuries or concussions. She sustained her first concussion as a freshman in college, after she was dropped while running through an advanced, and new, stunt during practice. Johnson fell hard, landing on her neck and head. She was scared by the fall and luckily did not sustain any spinal injuries. The concussion, and then post-concussive side effects, forced her to miss the rest of her first season. She then regained her health and returned to cheerleading.

But the memories of the fall and being shaken by it taught Johnson some valuable lessons. She says she will be telling every younger cheerleader she coaches at camps about the biggest thing she learned: Listen to your gut. She admits she didn't want to rock the boat, thinking that even asking a question of a coach or for asking for a few more run-throughs of a stunt at a slower speed would make her stick out as a troublemaker or a poor teammate. She also believed questioning would somehow let down her teammates or make her be viewed as less of a star cheerleader who could tackle anything.

These are all things she now knows she invented in her own mind, stemming from not having enough confidence and maturity to respectfully state her thoughts and concerns.

"I think that little feeling you get, knowing something is not right with you, or what you are about to do, is so important," Johnson says. "Doubt is not a bad thing. I think it is your heart and brain telling you to think an extra second about what you are doing. If you are not sure you should be doing some stunt you are not ready for, or if you are worried that your teammates may not be ready to catch you where they should, say something. Speak up, and tell a coach that you are unsure or have questions. Just going with it because you don't want to upset your teammates or have the coach not think you are awesome is not the way to go. It shows more responsibility to ask than to be 'brave' and get hurt. Please say something if you know you feel something isn't right. You'll never regret that."

LETTING OTHERS KNOW

But how can youth athletes let a coach or teammate know when they think they might have a serious injury? How can they say they are scared or that they think they may have gotten a concussion in an appropriate manner during a big moment in a game or competition? All children, no matter their age, understand pain and can express in their own words if and how something hurts. Having a supportive atmosphere, where youth athletes know they can tell the truth about how they feel and not be punished for expressing their fears, is critically important.

Dr. Christopher Giza, whom we met in Chapter 2, sees a big cultural change developing in youth sports both in his clinical work as a pediatric neurologist and in his experience as a parent. The word that concussions are something to be taken seriously is even filtering down to children, who are asking their own questions.

"I think it is important that athletes, even young ones, know . . . that they need to be part of the dialogue about concussions," Giza says. "They need to be able to know it is OK to say their head hurts, their vision seems different, or they feel sick to their stomachs. Those are all valuable diagnostic clues.

"Taking away any stigma about . . . mention[ing] concussion is important, and needs to be stated clearly by coaches and parents. Youth athletes that feel empowered to tell the truth will probably do so."

Still, even when everyone has the best of intentions going into a season, a game, or even a practice, it can be difficult for players to open up about fears, concerns, or symptoms. In addition to the issues discussed above, we cannot forget that people who are concussed may not possess the mental capacity to understand that they are injured, let alone communicate it.

For all of these reasons, it's extremely important to be proactive, not only reactive. Athletes of all ages, especially those who play contact sports, would do well to prepare for the possibility of being concussed. This preparation starts with education, of course, but it also requires developing good avenues of communication between all parties involved and having a concussion action plan in mind.

Unfortunately, it can be difficult to sort through the mountains of information and misinformation out there. My recommendation is to be leery of television productions, movies, or presentations in other media that have been produced for shock value. That's not to say that you can't trust anybody on TV or in the media, but certainly nobody deserves your trust just for being on there either. In the end, ask yourself what motivations you think people have for getting their message out and also question their sources of information.

You've already taken one very positive step: reading this book! The science and medicine of concussion are changing at a fast pace, however, so as a companion to this book I suggest that you visit the website concussionclarity.com for updated information. There are also plenty of good resources available from nonprofit organizations and professional societies. Some of these are listed in the section "Resources to Learn More About Sports Concussion" at the end of the book.

During your journey of concussion education, you should always strive to develop a good basic understanding of concussion and how it is different from PCS. Developing an appreciation for the "myth of simplicity" is also a great idea: Explore the ways in which each concussion is different, each person is different, and the reasons why there is no simple test for concussion diagnosis. Your goal should be to know as much about concussion (if not more!) than your coach.

Then, when you feel that you have a basic understanding of the issues, talk to people about it. Ask how your coach would respond if he or she thought you were concussed. Talk to your teammates or parents, and especially your athletic trainer if your team has one. That way, everybody will have at least talked about and will be more likely to be on the same page about how to recognize concussion and PCS, how these things are diagnosed, and how they're best managed.

Finally, have a plan for what to do if you get a concussion. Think through the entire process. Consider different possible scenarios and locations. Make sure your team has a plan for letting parents know about a concussion if they're not present. Where should you be taken if there are urgent concerns? Does your school have a plan for making academic accommodations to help you heal and to make sure that your academic ability is not unfairly judged while your brain is hurt?

Perhaps the most important part of any plan is identifying your local concussion healthcare providers. Where are these places located? Knowing and having quick access to phone numbers, office hours, and insurance needs are important too. Figuring these things out in advance can help recovery move along effectively.

But be cautious. Concussion clinics are popping up at a rapid rate all over the country. Not all these clinics are created equal, unfortunately. Do a little research into medical facilities that claim expertise in managing concussion. What types of professional clinicians do they have available? Do they operate under the medical supervision of a physician? As I'm sure you've figured out by now, concussion diagnosis and management can be quite complicated, often involving many confounding medical factors. Decisions about concussion care are medical ones that should be made by individuals who have the training and experience to consider the entire spectrum of brain health.

REFERENCES

1. Branch J. A snowboarder's dream and a family's anguish. *New York Times.* January 4, 2010. http://www.nytimes.com/2010/01/05/sports/olympics/05pearce.html.
2. ESPN Action Sports. Sarah Burke dies from injuries. January 20, 2012. http://xgames.espn.go.com/skiing/article/7466421/sarah-burke-dies-injuries-suffered-utah.

EIGHT

THOUGHTS FOR PARENTS
AND COACHES

Sports play a big part in our lives today, seemingly interwoven into all the strands that make up the complex fabric of society. Couples get engaged and married at sports stadiums. Babies can be clad from head to toe in outfits bearing the logos of sports teams.

And participating in sports, even at the youngest ages, serves as a rite of passage. Being athletic, especially through playing in some kind of group or team, can provide a lifetime's worth of treasured childhood memories. Sports can build character, discipline, and even courage that will serve the youth athlete well later in life. Sports bring joy, excitement, the health benefits of exercise, the mental and emotional challenges of competition, and, of course, a few bumps, bruises, and tears.

So we are surrounded by the sporting experience and culture, even if we don't see ourselves as the next NBA All-Star—or as the parent of one.

It's natural for parents—the audience to whom this chapter is largely addressed—to want to protect their kids from harm or danger and to want them to flourish and not suffer in any way. Our society is dramatically evolving to focus on the health and safety of playing sports. Our understanding of what may harm children when playing sports is greater, thanks to ongoing scientific research and changing attitudes.

Things that didn't happen in my childhood are now routine, even legally mandated. We place our kids in car seats from the moment they leave the hospital as newborns. Adults routinely wear seat belts while riding in cars, modeling safer behavior and following the law for their kids. Children are served healthier or organic foods, and we're keenly aware of life-threatening allergies to tree nuts. We're encouraged to be watchful about childhood obesity and the health issues created by sugar-laden or highly processed foods. We make sure to slather our children with sunscreen and to avoid sunburns to prevent skin cancer. Wearing helmets while riding bikes, skiing, or skateboarding is now the expectation more often than not.

Those are all pretty significant changes from the experiences of anybody born before the 1990s. Our parents also cared about our welfare, but societal standards and our awareness of childhood safety and health were clearly different.

SEEKING MIDDLE GROUND

It stands to reason, then, that care and concern for the welfare of youth athletes would also be at the top of our minds. Participation in childhood sports and organized team athletics has boomed since the 1980s, as more girls have gotten involved thanks to Title IX and our culture has become more sports-centric. Maybe you were an athlete as a child, and maybe you were talented and driven enough to play in high school, in college, or as part of an elite club.

We become hardwired through our own childhood experiences, and often we continue to play off those examples to form our parenting and coaching styles. We want to do better for our kids, and we want them to lead happy, successful, and fulfilling lives. Some of us see our kids as having the athletic potential to get athletic scholarships for college, become professional athletes, or participate in the Olympics. At the same time, to judge from growing survey data, we are becoming increasingly fearful that concussions from sports could endanger our children's health.

The desire for athletic success and the fear of injury are in opposition. To be blindly driven by either extreme would be counterproductive and ultimately harmful to our children and, I would argue, society at large. We need to have a rational discussion to find the middle ground between being too fearful and not being properly diligent about injury.

Right now, however, the extremes are the loudest voices in the national conversation about concussion in youth sports. We're either hearing denials that concussion is a serious issue that needs to be properly addressed—the "just a knock to the head" attitude—or fears of concussion so excessive that they make us want to keep our kids completely out of a sport such as football.

Of course, the path to common sense is not helped when parents read stories like a highly clicked-on 2015 article in Minneapolis' major newspaper, the *Star Tribune*, discussing two local doctors who recommended that football be eliminated from all schools to protect children.[1] These doctors maintained that the pressure to conform to the role of an athlete or to promote social status within a school community leads students to choose to play football over avoiding concussion risks. They were concerned that youth athletes are not in a position to understand or consent to the risks of playing football at any level. Ironically, in the second sentence of the *Star Tribune* article, one of the doctors—a bioethicist—is said to have admitted that an "outright ban on youth football would be unrealistic."

That brings us to living in the land of the real. There are many caring, well-meaning people on both sides of the concussion conversation, trying to do what is best for our youth athletes. I talk to them every day. Little by little I am starting to see a stripping away of the extreme positions, even as many national "experts" continue to drive their own agendas. I'm hopeful that in the end, accurate information and critical thought will win the day, bringing the two extremes together. What I work for every day is to advocate for and consciously move the conversation to the middle ground—a more thoughtful, science-based view of the role of sports in our kids' lives. Being a supportive sports parent is important, because you set the tone for your child's experience. Being afraid of concussion or overly protective to the point of making nearly everything scary will imprint itself onto your child. And the other extreme, the mindset that your child can just play through a concussion and act like nothing is wrong, is equally problematic.

INCREASED PARENTAL AWARENESS

Sarah Clark has pretty much seen it all as an involved mom of two athletic sons who played football, baseball, and basketball at Skyline High School in Ann Arbor, Michigan. Her oldest son, Jack, sustained three concussions in five years. His first occurred in 2009, during a football play in his freshman year. Jack's second concussion happened a year later, when he was at a basketball camp and was popped in the head by an elbow during a scrimmage. His final concussion happened while playing college baseball as a freshman, when he was hit in the face by the bad skip of a grounder. Clark now jokes that Jack spaced his injuries at the pace of one per sport.

Jack returned to play after each concussion, thanks to proper treatment and dynamic return-to-play protocols. Clark did her homework too, trying to learn about concussions and the recovery process. All three of Jack's concussions healed successfully, and he continued to play sports without further issues. He now plays varsity baseball at Kalamazoo College.

Clark's younger son, Willy, is 2015 high school graduate who played varsity basketball and football. Willy now plays halfback for the varsity football team at Carnegie Mellon University. He is bigger than Jack and is a more physical and bruising player in basketball and football than his older brother. Still, Clark says she is confident in the university's concussion protocols and trainers to keep him safe.

Clark says she has watched attitudes toward concussion among parents swing from one side to the other since 2009. She sees parents keeping their sons out of football because they are worried about the perception of lasting negative health effects of concussions. Clark takes in their tales but doesn't let them sway her approach to parenting. She understands their concerns, because she too is a parent who wants to protect her children—even if her once little boys are now grown into tall, strong men.

"I don't think I was ever that super-worried, hovering-over-my-kids mom, even before Jack got his first concussion. I understand that injuries happen and I wasn't going to stop my boys from playing football or anything else like that in sports," Clark says. "What has changed over the past few years, now that we are really talking about concussions, is that there is so much confusion out there about what a concussion is. We're aware of it, but I think because we can't see a concussion or check on how it is healing, it makes some parents afraid. We don't know how to assess it. We don't how it gets fixed.

"If Jack had a sprained ankle, I could say, 'Wow, it really looks purple or swollen' or go look at an X-ray and see that his bone is broken. We, as parents, can see and understand that even if we're not doctors. But I can't look inside my boys' heads and see that something is wrong after they've been hit, and I think that's the real root of the issue and why some parents are scared."

Clark's involvement as a sports parent at the school led her to become the president of the athletic booster club in 2014. Now that she is part of the formal process running sports at Skyline High, she sees ways for parents to become involved in the concussion awareness discussion at their schools and clubs. She works with the school's athletic director, along with her fellow members of the booster club, to ensure that reasonable and open dialogue about concussions takes place among the school administration, coaches, athletic trainers, parents, and athletes. She says she saw the benefits of the growing openness about the topic when a few athletes during the fall 2014 season told athletic trainers and coaches that they or a teammate might have sustained a concussion.

Pete Vaz, a longtime and successful high school basketball coach in the Fremont, California area, has seen the same kinds of changes in concussion awareness as Clark. Vaz, whom we first met in Chapter 2, admits he never thought of concussion as an injury that he should be concerned about in nearly three decades of coaching prep camps for basketball and running. Sprained ankles, broken fingers, and even knee injuries were higher on his list of concerns. Players sometimes accidentally took blows to the head when rebounding or playing down low. If they seemed OK or wanted to keep playing, Vaz usually didn't stand in their way. He figured that if something were really wrong, they'd say something. Or maybe they'd shake off the cobwebs and show their toughness and dedication by continuing to play.

But now he doesn't allow players who've been hit this way to continue to play or practice until they are evaluated for possible concussion. Vaz says he makes sure the school trainer, his coaching staff, players, and athletic trainers are continuously watchful. He seeks out information on concussions and wants to find the best way to walk the line between safety and building strong and smart players.

"It's not that we didn't care, or that we were trying to be tough, we just didn't know," says Vaz, who is also a teacher. "It really is crazy to think of how far we have come in talking about this in such a short time. Nobody talked about concussions 5 or 10 years ago—not the parents, not the trainers, and definitely not the kids. Now it seems like not a day goes by when it isn't being brought up in some way. I think it's good that we are more aware. We just try to keep things in perspective if we can."

TAKING
ON PRODUCTIVE ROLES

A doctor's visit can be uncomfortable or unsettling, because it usually occurs when something is wrong. Patients normally don't come see me when their brains are working well or if they are feeling great. That would be a less tense appointment! Patients and their parents are coming in to see me because something has happened during a game or practice and they need an evaluation. They are worried that something is really wrong.

There's usually a characteristic set of people sitting in my examination room: the athlete and a parent or two. The athlete is nervous, wondering what the exam is going to be like and what is going to happen as a result. The parents are also nervous, even a bit anxious, trying to anticipate what's wrong or how bad it could be. Sometimes the parents and athlete have Googled their symptoms and come to their own conclusions based on what they found at various websites, in social media postings, and in archived news reports. That array of information, usually flying around their thoughts without context or medical confirmation, quite often adds to their anxiety.

Despite the uneasy vibe in the room, the right things are happening. Seeing the appropriate medical professional after a concussion is a critical step that enables the patient to be properly assessed, tested, and monitored. Pediatricians and family practice physicians can be great for starting the process of dealing with a concussion, but seeing a neurologist often leads to more effective diagnosis and management, especially in more complex cases. Regardless, it's important that care providers taking care of concussions have a comprehensive and critical approach to neurological diagnosis and management.

Parents want to hear that their children will be fine and will return to good health. Athletes usually want to hear that they will soon get back to playing their sports and hanging with their teammates. More often than not, I see happy outcomes, which is great. I too am rooting for a happy ending for my patients.

Parents play important roles in concussion prevention and safety, from understanding their school's or team's protocols and policies to knowing where to go and what to do in case of a concussion to remaining vigilant—and positive—during the recovery phase.

Clark recommends that parents also consider that their child's coaches are not like professional or elite coaches. Most youth and prep coaches are unpaid volunteers or are reimbursed only nominally for their time. They get involved in coaching to be with their children, for love of the school where they work, or to be part of the community. Sometimes a parent is drafted into coaching duty and says yes out of love for his or her child. Most youth and prep coaches are doing the best they can. Their good intentions are undoubtable.

Clark also thinks it is a good idea to get a sense of how your child's coaches do their jobs and of what the athletes are doing in practices. Just don't be an intrusion, trying to conduct an on-the-spot grand jury investigation into how the coaches run things.

"I say this in a general way, and not to rock the boat, but as parents of kids in sports, especially the lower-level ones where they may just be starting out, you can't be sure that the coaches know any more than you do about concussions," Clark says. "A lot of them are just volunteers or not really getting paid a lot, so their being coaches doesn't automatically mean they are trained on how to best deal with concussions. I think you can do a lot of good by watching a practice, or having your athletic director pop in on some, to see what the coaches are doing and how the players are looking out there. If you see something that looks dangerous or not totally right, it's good for the proper channels, like the booster club or athletic director, to know."

Clark cautions parents, from experience, not to be backseat drivers to the coaches. That's a great way to cause friction, and the rifts that result can cause significant issues for the team. Instead, she encourages parents to use the resources of the athletic program or club, such as the athletic director, parent representatives, athletic trainers, or booster boards, to make sure that problematic safety issues get discussed with coaches.

BEING PROPERLY PROTECTIVE

Kate Markgraf, whom we last met in Chapter 7, is retired from soccer but remains in the sports world as a mom to three active young children who are involved in ice hockey and soccer. Football, however, is out for her two sons, because she is concerned about the potential for injury.

"My kids play sports, and if something happens like a concussion, I hope I have enough awareness to make the right decisions, and I definitely will watch for any lingering side effects," Markgraf says. "I have really rough kids. They are wrestling all the time, flying around the house. So they're definitely active, and there is silliness and love in our house."

While Markgraf obviously cannot turn off being an expert on soccer when she is standing on the sidelines during her children's games, she says she chooses to let their coaches do the teaching and development without any interference from her. She has, however, instituted one firm rule about how she wants her kids to play while they are under the age of 14: no headers. Her stance is echoed by her former US National Team teammates Brandi Chastain and Cindy Parlow-Cone, who have come out against heading by youth soccer players in a national campaign.

Change is in fact coming to youth soccer in the United States. A lawsuit filed against US Soccer, the United States Youth Soccer Association, the American Youth Soccer Organization, US Club Soccer, and the California Youth Soccer Association was settled in August 2015.[2] Part of the resulting agreement calls for recommending that children under the age of 10 be barred from heading the ball and that players between 11 and 13 be limited to only heading during practice. Additionally, the substitution rules were modified to allow any player who is suspected to be concussed to get an in-game evaluation without penalty to the team.

These changes result from organized soccer's looking into how the contact parts of the game could affect children and are part of the sport's evolving stance on concussions.

For her part, Markgraf does not think it is necessary for her children to practice headers or execute them in a game to progress in youth soccer. She believes that her rule may spare them unnecessary brain trauma while they are young and help them to develop other important soccer skills, like bringing the ball under control with their chest. Her sons love to take corner kicks, and she is fine with that for their level of youth soccer.

"I don't see them missing out on anything by not heading yet," says Markgraf. "I won't even practice headers with them in the backyard. They know not to even ask. I feel that strongly about it. When they are older and their brains are more developed, we can look at it again. But for now, no headers until they are 14."

Markgraf helps coach elite girls' soccer clubs in Wisconsin and hears a lot about players on these teams being out of action thanks to concussions. Seeing what is happening at the youth level, along with her experiences, has driven her thought process about headers.

"I'd rather err on the side of caution," she says, "but I also don't have any hard, strict rules. I'm not going to take my kids out of sports, nothing that extreme. It's something they love. We're going to be smart about what we do."

Markgraf says she also keeps an eye on her three children when they play ice hockey, wanting to encourage proper technique and body awareness. Her oldest son used to run into the boards to stop himself, because his skating skills weren't yet up to par. She says she told him that he had to work on stopping properly, without risking going head first into the boards, or he would not move up. With some practice, he soon figured out how to stop, and she allowed him to advance a level.

HELPING CHILDREN ADMIT THEY'RE HURT

Andy Murray has seen all three of his children—two sons and a daughter—turn their ice hockey talent into their professions. He's been through the early morning weekend practices; he's seen them play on high school, juniors', and college teams; and now they're on professional teams in Switzerland. He also well understands the coaching side, having been the head coach of the NHL's Los Angeles Kings and St. Louis Blues, the general manager of Team Canada, and now the head coach for Western Michigan University's hockey team.

Murray wants parents to approach concussion with a serious attitude, but not to the point where they remove contact sports from the options they will consider for their children. Ice hockey is certainly a physical game, and the widespread emphasis on toughness is part of the sport that he hopes can be reshaped a bit with improved concussion awareness. He says he maintained a strong relationship with his children as they learned the sport, emphasizing sportsmanship and injury awareness as much as stickhandling and checking.

"My kids went through having concussions, and I was obviously concerned, but I knew we were handling things correctly and in a timely fashion—we never denied what was happening," Murray says. "The attitude that was in hockey when I was coming up as a player was to never admit you were hurt. Never say anything is wrong, because then you aren't tough enough or you won't get to play again. I made sure my children knew not only did I expect them to be honest if they felt they were hurt; I encouraged them to do so as part of being a strong member of the team.

"Taking care of your body is part of being on the team. I never worried that they were trying to hide something from us or the coaches. I feel that made a big difference for them."

Establishing that mindset in your children can make all the difference. Yes, there is a fine line to be walked between enabling children to bring up possibly serious injuries and encouraging them to mention every single bump and scratch, especially for children who may not yet be mature enough to exercise proper judgment. A certain amount of resilience, determination, and pushing through discomfort is needed at times to play sports and be an effective athlete. Still, it's important to set up a standard for all children that honesty is the best policy and that the child should let a coach, athletic trainer, or parent know if something is wrong. Speaking up about feeling woozy, having a headache, or other symptoms of a possible concussion is necessary. And key to this is the child's knowing that their parents or coaches will not be mad at or disappointed in them if they do.

There are also gender differences to keep in mind when empowering a child athlete to discuss injuries. Studies tell us that females tend to report concussions more than males. There could be several reasons for this disparity: Females tend to be more verbal and better at discussing what is going on with their symptoms. Culturally, it is more possible for female athletes to admit they are hurt without being perceived as being weak. This is not to say that female athletes, who can be every bit as tough and stubborn as male athletes at all levels, may not choose to ignore an injury and try to play through it.

Males, on the other hand, tend more than females to face the burden that denying and avoiding weakness is often seen as central to being "tough." This is especially true in predominantly male sports such as football. Being injured or thinking you might be injured then puts you into the category of being "weak." Even worse, old-school coaches, including some famous examples, have used vulgar terms that play off male anxieties about gender and sexual identity as code words for not being tough enough or being "soft."

Thankfully, society has largely grown to view harshly assessing injury as weakness as both untrue and demeaning. Many of the best athletes, from Olympic gold medal–winning skier Lindsey Vonn to one of the toughest and greatest athletes of all time, boxer Muhammad Ali, suffered significant injuries while competing that they did not hide from the public. The world certainly does not regard Vonn or Ali as "weak" or "whiners." They are thought of as champions who worked hard and were the best in their sports.

Still, even when there is a supportive family and coaching system in place, a child may find it a difficult challenge to take the initiative to say that something is wrong, especially if it is serious.

Eric Hipple's 15-year-old son, Jeff, who never played a down of organized football or any other contact sport and never had a concussion, ended up in the same cycle of fighting depression that his father had gone through (see Chapter 6). Jeff wasn't open about how he felt, and Hipple says he didn't push Jeff to open up. So Jeff successfully hid his mental and emotional pain. Sadly, he ended his life through suicide in 2000. Losing his son and enduring feelings of guilt, grief, and powerlessness over his death have given Hipple a different perspective on life.

"I now realize things were not right with my son, even though I thought they were or hoped they were," says Hipple, now an advocate for facing depression and preventing suicide among teens. "I used sports and being a good athlete to try to hide what was wrong with me. That didn't work.

"My son ended up in the same place. He withdrew and became more reclusive than I was as a kid, but it was the same place. I tell parents, if you think something is going on, don't let it go. We don't want to think something serious is going on, or that our children are depressed or struggling. Something like a concussion could set that off, and we need to be aware.

I will always wonder what I could have done to help Jeff if I had known then what I know now. I will think about that until the day I die."

For all these reasons, it's important to give our sons and daughters the permission and freedom to tell their coaches, athletic trainers, and us that they are feeling bad or strange or that a teammate could be injured. Being honest about concussions is a sign of true strength and of being a positive teammate.

THE IMPORTANCE OF JUST BEING THERE

In Chapter 7 we met snowboarder Ellery Hollingsworth. Hollingsworth's mother, Linherr, has always tried to protect her fearless daughter from sports injury. She was with Hollingsworth every step of the way as she built her snowboarding career. Linherr finds it a bit ironic that she moved her daughter out of ice hockey and into skiing when Hollingsworth was around age 8 or 9, thinking snow would be a safer place. She was worried about Hollingsworth falling or getting knocked over as a slight girl playing hockey mostly with boys. Little did Linherr know the hard falls that her daughter would endure while developing into an elite snowboarder.

As a mom, Linherr says she learned to balance her concerns with the realities of her daughter's chosen sport. She emphasized safety to Hollingsworth, outfitted her with a helmet early on, and made sure to check in to see how she really was feeling after a rough day of training or competition. Top snowboarders are naturally tough, sometimes bordering on unreasonably fearless.

"I didn't want Ellery to hide things from me if she was hurt, even though I know now that she did," Linherr says. "It was hard to see the falls sometimes. I could feel that it had to hurt. She got checked out, and if they said she was fine and she wanted to go again, she went. Still, we were worried."

As Hollingsworth's career took off, she was less often at home surrounded by family. She was out competing and training around the world, and Linherr had to trust coaches and athletic trainers to take care of her daughter. Things came full circle at the end of Hollingsworth's career, when she needed her family's help to overcome a serious concussion and, later, significant post-concussive issues.

"When she had that last concussion, and her personality changed into being down and depressed, we were there for her," Linherr says. "No question. I know having that closeness made the difference, because we were there to help her when she needed it."

Hollingsworth admits that at her career's end, when she was suffering from post-concussive issues, it was hard to fully turn to her family for help in recovering. She reluctantly moved home for a while, surrendering some independence, but eventually she healed.

"It was super hard moving back home and asking my parents for help, but it was the right thing to do," Hollingsworth says. "Having that loving and real relationship with my parents, which has always been there since I was a kid, helped me admit I needed to focus on getting better. My family has always been there for me, from the start, when I was a kid, to the middle, when I was competing, to the end."

WHAT COACHES CAN DO

Till now we've been largely talking about the roles parents can play in promoting concussion awareness and safety. Now let's consider what contributions coaches can make.

It's obvious that not all youth sports coaches use the same approaches or even have similar reasons for participation. There is the dad or mom who is an assistant softball coach for their daughter's third-grade team, on the staff more for support than to create the next pitching star like Olympian Jennie Finch. There are the parents who coach their child in the same sport they excelled in when they were young, bringing a more competitive and honed point of view to their coaching. And then there are the coaches who are lifers, successfully coaching and mentoring team after team long after their own children have graduated.

No matter where you are in the coaching spectrum, there are some things you can do to make your time more effective from a concussion awareness standpoint. Hopefully you will develop close relationships with the players by being around them. Knowing their personalities, understanding how they think, and having a feel for what is normal behavior for your youth athletes are important for detecting when they are behaving abnormally—a clue to a possible concussion.

Coaches walk a fine line between advocating a useful level of toughness and discipline during play and leading athletes to believe they should play through injury or pain. They should help youth athletes understand the important distinction between a harmless scrape and a significant second of wooziness. Passing along this lesson may be challenging when the athletes are younger, as emotional and mental maturity may affect their perceptions of how hurt they are.

Emphasizing telling the truth is important at every stage. Studies are increasingly revealing that youth athletes are open to lying or otherwise deceiving their coaches and athletic trainers about being concussed. There is even growing research indicating that some athletes try to game baseline testing to register a lower score. They think that performing poorly on the baseline test will help them get back to playing sooner if they are concussed. How would that work? If they get a poor score on a test performed post-concussion and it is compared to an artificially lowered baseline, the difference will be smaller than if they'd had an honest baseline score. They assume that with a small enough difference, they will be cleared to play—even though they will in fact be concussed. It's an unwise move but can seem logical to an athlete who wants to keep playing at any cost.

The reality is, when physicians are evaluating a patient for concussion and figuring out a return-to-play plan, it's not that hard to see when somebody has performed poorly on their baseline test on purpose. The natural clinical instinct is then to be more conservative about that patient's return, since the patient now seems like someone who'll be deceptive about how they're doing during recovery. As a result, the athlete ends up being out of play longer than if they had given the baseline testing their best effort.

A notion I've heard from athletes who think being evasive about injury is a smart ploy is that being concussed means that not only are they coming out of a game but they possibly will not play again. They worry that they'll lose their starting roles, that their scholarships or recruiting status will be compromised, and that their coaches will view them as damaged goods.

HAVING THE COURAGE TO BE SAFE

Murray wants to redefine the concept of admitting injury as being a bad thing at all levels of ice hockey. He admits that his sport has historically not treated injuries, especially to the head, with adequate seriousness. He has been in the game long enough to remember the days of NHL players competing without helmets and of goalies facing blistering slap shots without any facial or cranial protection. Legendary Montreal Canadiens goalie Jacques Plante created a stir on November 1, 1959, when he became the first goalie to wear a mask in a regular-season game.[3] Today, putting a player at any level on the ice without a helmet or full goalie gear would seem shocking.

Both equipment and concussion awareness have improved dramatically in hockey, but Murray still finds a bit of resistance to changing its warrior mentality. Hockey is a rough sport in which professional players are celebrated for being bloodied, taking a quick hit of stitches, and then returning to play in the same game.

But to Murray as a coach, and also as a mentor and father figure for his college players, anything short of being totally responsible and accountable about brain health is unacceptable for his team. He does not praise players who take risks, on or off the ice, and he has a no-tolerance policy for concussions. The health of his hockey players comes first, and then the business of hopefully winning games and championships.

"As coaches, we are the leaders who have to communicate what the core beliefs of our team are from the start: We do not play hockey in an unsafe or dangerous manner or any other way that harms our players or opponents," Murray says. "That probably sounds like it should be a little obvious, but I don't think it is, from my experience at all levels of hockey. We take concussions seriously. Nobody on our team will knowingly be playing with a concussion, or trying to come back to play while they are in recovery mode.

"We communicate that at the start of the season as a coaching staff; our athletic training staff says the same; I tell players we are recruiting the same; and I tell their parents the same thing. We are very clear on that message. There is no heroism or credit given for playing through a concussion. It's unwise, it's dangerous, and we do not knowingly allow it to happen."

Murray would like to see the same no-tolerance message delivered throughout hockey, with a special focus on youth, minor, and junior leagues. From stories he hears and things he has witnessed, he feels there may be more risk-taking allowed at those levels as players seek to make a name for themselves. If Murray had his way, youth players would be taught clear lessons on how to take care of their health in every league and camp. He thinks mandated concussion education for players, coaches, parents, host families, and leagues would make hockey a safer sport.

"We're doing a lot, and things have progressed for sure, but there is a lot more we can do to make hockey smarter about concussions," Murray says. "The awareness is getting up there, but making sure the practices are everywhere and players don't feel they need to hide things to get ahead will make even more change. I don't want any of my players to get concussions, but I know it is going to happen because of what the game of hockey is.

"The question then becomes, how can we be smarter about getting our players the concussion treatment they need and helping them continue their careers or lives in a good manner? That is what I want all of us in hockey to focus on."

Murray has made an effort to become educated about concussions and to work with his athletic training staff and team doctors to ensure they are all on the same page. I think the same approach is critical for coaches at all levels. You may not have the same resources as Murray, who coaches at a Division I school with an established hockey program, but you can likely tap into other support systems around you for concussion education.

Many youth leagues and school systems are mandating that coaches go through some sort of training in basic first aid, coaching and management techniques, and other useful tools for running a team. Hopefully your training program is up to date and discusses concussions, including signs that one may have occurred. Hopefully your school also has established and disseminated clear protocols for dealing with suspected concussion. If your training does not or did not discuss concussion, ask your league manager or school athletic director if other resources are available. If your school has an athletic trainer, make sure you have a good working relationship and know the trainer's concussion protocol. The trainer may not be able to cover every practice or game because of availability and the need to cover multiple sports, but having a good understanding of what the trainer needs to know in case of injury can be helpful to you if he or she isn't around. Developing a formal concussion protocol, but filing it away in a cabinet with nobody understanding it doesn't work.

Especially at the beginner levels, the coach or assistants may be the first ones to suspect that a concussion has occurred. You thus may be the critical link in determining if a player should come out to be assessed. Having the courage to make the right decision—which is to sit a player out if you have any suspicion of concussion—is paramount. There should be no distinction in this matter between a star player and a reserve, between the final minutes of a championship game and a preseason blowout, or between a game, a practice, and some goofing around during pickup play. If you spot something that suggests an athlete is concussed, if the athlete is acting strangely or showing other concussion symptoms, you have to be the voice of reason and responsibility. Hopefully there will be an athletic trainer on site to help you at that moment, but if not, the first step is taking the athlete out of the game or practice until he or she can be properly evaluated by a medical professional.

Coaches aren't perfect. Parents aren't perfect. Players aren't perfect. Sports serve as an emotional crucible, in which we ride on waves of joy, tension, and, sometimes, sadness. But determining if an athlete is concussed shouldn't be an emotional decision.

It should be the right decision.

REFERENCES

1. Olson J. Minnesota doctors call for removal of football from public schools. *Minneapolis Star Tribune*. November 21, 2015. http://www.startribune.com/minnesota-doctors-call-for-removal-of-football-from-public-schools/352464821/.
2. US Soccer. Joint statement regarding concussion lawsuit resolution. November 2, 2015. http://www.ussoccer.com/about/recognize-to-recover/concussion-guidelines/player-safety-campaign-faqs.
3. Roarke SP. Playing without mask unthinkable to today's goalies. October 28, 2009. http://www.nhl.com/ice/news.htm?id=503855.

NINE

CHANGING THE GAME,
ON AND OFF THE FIELD

Clearly there are a lot of issues swirling around sports concussion. Increased awareness and concern are leading to rule changes across the sports landscape at every level of play. Numerous businesses are stepping in, hawking products to address concussion awareness or treatment, tests to "instantly" diagnose concussions on the sideline, devices to measure concussions, alternative ways to "heal" concussions, and even ways to "repair" the damage done to the brain. A lot of the advertising for these products is pitched to parents and youth coaches; it's smart business to target a potential customer base representing the roughly 46.5 million child athletes in US organized sports. And the sales pitch isn't that hard—parents usually want to do anything in their power to keep their children safe and properly equipped, sometimes even if it is unproven. Many of these treatments, services, or products require a significant financial commitment.

Expensive, experimental, or not, it can be challenging to figure out what products to consider and to look critically at them given how incomplete the science around concussions is.

In every case, I urge patients, families, and clinicians to pay attention to whether any scientific evidence supports—or perhaps argues against—the effectiveness and safety of the products they're considering buying, and what that evidence consists of. Prevention of injury is obviously a key focus of products and services and needs to be the subject of stronger scientific inquiry. Another hot area is the use of baseline testing for concussion management, and each test comes with its own body of evidence.

The number of products addressing sports concussion is growing and expanding every day. Let's look at what's out there now, and what factors one should pay closer attention to when considering spending money on these products.

WHAT HELMETS CAN AND CANNOT DO

The first line of defense against a concussion that most people would think of is a helmet. The first mention of football helmets in the media dates back to 1893, when Joseph Mason Reed reportedly had a moleskin hat with earflaps made to prevent damage from getting kicked in the head.[1] By the 1920s, the soft leather hat–helmet had turned into a harder design. Plastic helmets were introduced a decade later, and by the 1940s they were mandatory equipment for college and NFL players. Additions such as face masks, ear holes, air vents, and foam padding inside the helmets were some of the next design improvements. More recent advances in materials science and energy management designs have continued to push the helmet design envelope.

Regardless of the sport, helmets have evolved a lot and will continue to do so. They are clearly now high-tech gear, with some youth football helmets costing upwards of $300. Helmets for other sports, such as ice hockey, field hockey, lacrosse, and skiing, commonly run $100 or more. There is certainly a good reason for their being expensive. No area of sports safety is more critical than protecting the brain, and the engineering and materials necessary to address this goal can be costly.

It's clear why helmets are useful. First and foremost, they protect the skull from injury. And protect the skull means protect the brain, right? Not necessarily. A helmet in fact cannot completely protect the brain from concussion. That's a consequence of the underlying mechanism of injury. Think of the helmet as an eggshell, and the egg yolk as the brain. The eggshell protects the yolk from leaking out if a blow shakes it. But the eggshell does not protect what is inside it from moving around. Shake an egg, and the yolk will slosh around and possibly become damaged. A concussion occurs if a jolt is significant enough to jostle the brain, and a helmet has a limited ability to stop the forces responsible.

So the notion that a top-of-the-line helmet or the most expensive model will absolutely prevent concussion is false. That is not to say that helmets have no role in concussion prevention.

On the contrary, they are extremely important. Remember that what might be most important for long-term brain health is not how many concussions somebody has been diagnosed with but how much force the brain has experienced over one's life. A person's overall lifetime exposure to force is therefore something we should try to minimize. Going back to the image of the egg yolk and the eggshell, a good shell (the helmet) can lessen the amount of force the yolk (brain) experiences. So using a helmet that lets the least amount of force through to the brain from any given impact not only may reduce the number of concussions, even if it cannot prevent them completely, but it may have longer and deeper positive effects by preventing long-term neurological consequences of cumulative exposure to force.

Helmets won't stop every injury, and they were never meant to provide a magic shield from outside forces. Nonetheless, having a high-quality, correctly fitted helmet and wearing it properly for both athletic practice and competition is vitally important. A helmet definitely can provide important skull protection during accidents involving traumatic brain injury, like falling while skiing and hitting a hidden rock or tree stump.

Finding the right helmet, getting it fit so it sits properly on the head, and wearing it correctly (yes, that means having the chinstrap correctly secured around your chin) are important steps in protecting an athlete's brain. So is periodically assessing it for damage. Helmets are not indestructible, despite their hard appearance, high-tech designs, and advanced materials. I have witnessed helmets break firsthand many times, perhaps most notably at the 2014 Sochi Winter Olympics. While I was working as part of the US medical staff on duty at the women's slopestyle course, snowboard semifinals competitor Sarka Pancochova of the Czech Republic under-rotated after a jump, missed her usual landing, and fell awkwardly and violently. You might have seen this on the news or online, as the dramatic and scary video quickly went viral worldwide. She slammed into the snow hard, with her back, neck, and helmet taking the brunt of the collision. Her head hit the packed snow surface. She briefly lost consciousness and went limp from the impact. The world watched Pancochova slide down the rest of the course on her side and back like a rag doll. She quickly regained consciousness, but was clearly dazed at the bottom of the course. She took off her helmet in the judging/TV area, and the TV cameras zoomed in to gauge her reaction to the judges' scores. The low scores didn't shock her. Her face did, however, clearly register a surprised look when she found that the violent impact from her accident had split open the hard shell of her helmet.[2] Pancochova was OK and finished fifth in the Olympic competition. But imagine the damage that could have happened if her bare head had taken the primary force of that impact instead of her helmet.

So wearing a helmet for practice, play, or competition is important. Accidents can happen at any time, even if you're just out for a casual run down the slopes or a horseback ride.

We just need to remember that helmets have their limitations as protective devices.

HELMET SAFETY STANDARDS

The most referenced safety standards for helmets in the United States are created and maintained by the National Operating Committee on Standards for Athletic Equipment (NOCSAE), which was established in 1969. NOCSAE takes a sports-specific approach to examining helmets for many, but not all, sports. The organization's standards should be considered the bare minimum, not the gold standard, for protection. As helmets evolve along with our understanding of the dangers of head impacts, so should helmet standards. There have been recent calls for more stringent standards in individual sports and for making standards more specific to the types of impacts that are most likely to occur in a given sport. Standards are always changing, and you should take a moment when shopping for a helmet to make sure that the models you're considering have passed the most current requirements.

Many efforts, typically from the academic world, have been made to examine helmets from different manufacturers and compare the levels of protection they provide. Most of this research has examined different makes of football helmets. The most talked-about helmet rating system is STAR (Summation of Tests for the Analysis of Risk), developed by safety engineers at Virginia Tech. This evaluation system is based on a scale from one to five stars, with five being the highest rating and one the lowest. Results of testing specific helmets with the Virginia Tech STAR system are available online[3] and are usually updated as new helmet models come to market. To date, helmets for both ice hockey and football have been ranked with the STAR system.

Here are a few words of caution, however, about relying on these ratings. The STAR system is based on how helmets perform in a laboratory setting, where the amount of force a helmet lets through to the mechanical head wearing it is measured. This approach may be good for understanding the physics of the forces produced from sport-related contact. By varying the delivery of the force in the lab, the researchers can simulate different types of contact, such as running into the hockey boards off a check. But there is a huge difference between a mechanical head and a living brain. It is impossible to predict real injury rates or precisely describe injury severity by looking only at the mathematics of the physical insult. Brains don't work that way, and as you've learned, every injury is personal and unique. So when you see a STAR rating, you should realize that it reflects the helmet's mechanical abilities and not clinical measures.

To be clear, I certainly would like to see all my patients wear helmets that let the least amount of force through to the brain. Be smart and protect yourself. At the same time, be cautious about any claims of injury reduction that stem from a helmet's STAR rating.

The other word of caution I want to add about STAR ratings stems from the fact that they do not take into account variables that relate to the world of sports in particular. The engineers approach the safety problem in sports much as they would the study of other safety products, like automobile seat belts. It's possible to understand the physics of car crashes, human bodies, and mechanical restraints to a level that permits drawing conclusions about safety, allowing engineers to tell product designers ways to improve safety in the real world. But what if the type of seat belt you used affected your ability to drive the car safely? What if the materials used, the weight, the size, and so on actually made it easier or harder for you to change lanes or turn a corner? Of course, any real-world design would take these things into account.

In contact sports, however, helmets not only must provide an acceptable level of safety but must do so while having physical qualities that allow the athlete to interact with the sporting environment quickly and efficiently. I'm not saying that if given a choice, we should ever sacrifice safety for performance. But any rating of safety equipment that does not consider how the particular sport in question is played, by each position, by different age groups, and at different levels, is leaving out a very large part of what the rating needs to reflect.

A great example of this is ice hockey helmets. There is a widely held consensus that hockey helmets (and lacrosse helmets too) are not as protective as football helmets. There are two pretty obvious reasons for this difference. First, the number of impacts in football, and how and when they occur, is unique to that sport. Second, any athlete who tried to play ice hockey (or lacrosse) with a football helmet would have disadvantages with respect to movement and vision that would actually make them more vulnerable to injury.

So when I saw the results of the STAR system's testing of ice hockey helmets, I was not surprised that none of them received the five-star rating that was given to many football helmets. Hockey and football are completely different sports, with different athletic requirements. My main takeaway from those ratings was that there is no hockey helmet that should be recommended for playing football.

TIPS FOR HELMET BUYERS

A helmet can only provide proper protection if it fits correctly. In general, for football, hockey, and lacrosse helmets, you can start to get a good idea of fit by measuring the skull around the crown of the head and matching that to the size specifications of the particular helmet model. In most sports, the front of the helmet should sit about an inch or two above the brow, and the back of the skull should be covered down to the top of the neck. A helmet should not be so tight that it is uncomfortable, but it needs to be snug enough to prevent it from moving freely.

People in charge of equipment purchases should look for helmets that are durable, are made with high-quality materials, and pass all safety standards. If many models exist, the most expensive one isn't always the best or worth the extra money. Be wary about hand-me-down or secondhand helmets. They may not fit correctly, may have cracked shells or other forms of protective compromise, or may have poorly fitting or damaged padding on the inside. Most high school programs recondition helmets, getting professional companies to replace worn-out padding, sanitize any remaining interior surfaces, check for damage, and make sure the helmets still pass the basic standards. It's an added expense for schools and programs, but one that must be incurred to ensure safety. It's the right thing to do to protect players.

Passing the standards unfortunately does not always guarantee that the helmet is a good one. Late in 2014, NOCSAE voided the certification status of two popular helmet brands worn by youth, high school, and college lacrosse players because of safety concerns. Much like what we see with automobile recalls, updated safety information is issued about helmet models periodically. It's important to keep on top of such developments for the helmet or helmets you use—and even if they continue to be "officially" up to par, checking each helmet regularly for damage remains critical.

HELMETS AND BEHAVIOR

A problem I commonly see is parents' and athletes' drawing a false sense of security from helmets. The danger is that helmet use may actually make athletes more aggressive, because they feel that donning armor-like protective equipment means they will not be injured. We actually see this with other protective equipment. In ice hockey, for example, the shoulder pads and elbow pads have become so good at protecting the wearer, not only from injury but also from feeling any pain when delivering a check, that many observers feel the physicality of the sport has increased to unsafe levels.

Let's take a closer look at the idea that "armoring up" players in more protective equipment might be having a negative effect on overall sport safety. According to a theory called "risk compensation," people adjust their behavior to reflect their perception of danger. Thus players wearing helmets and other protective equipment may play more aggressively because the additional level of protection from injury makes them feel more indestructible. They also may be less mindful of their opponents' safety, because they feel all athletes in the game are injury-proofed by the layers of equipment.

This concept is gaining more traction, especially in American football and ice hockey circles. It used to be normal practice for football players to lead tackles with their heads or to launch themselves horizontally at other players, essentially using their bodies as battering rams—a maneuver known as spearing. Practice schemes such as the infamous "Oklahoma" drill often led to injury when players were directed to collide at full speed, because they involved unwarranted levels of aggression and helmet-to-helmet contact. Thankfully, these practices have largely been discredited at all levels, as players suffered head, neck, and back damage from the violent collisions. Moreover, these "tests" of toughness often backfired: Injured players meant depleted rosters.

More and more, sports leagues are actively responding to such overly aggressive behavior. Recent years have seen the adoption of new prohibitions and higher penalties for spearing or deliberate head-to-head contact to discourage players from leading with their heads. With these changes, we should be able to figure out how the psychological theories compare with the statistical reality.

Could better helmets (or the use of helmets or other head protection in traditionally "non-helmeted" sports) lead to more injury? Possibly. The counterargument comes from people who compare that prediction with another prediction from risk compensation theory: that wearing seat belts would lead to higher rates of unsafe driving. Statistical evidence shows, however, that using seat belts actually saves lives. Whatever the reality is, it's clear that each sport has its own set of things to consider.

Risk compensation theory also leads to the interesting prediction that *less* protective equipment might actually lead to more careful play. Some social science researchers have begun looking into this question. Late in the 2014 season, a National Public Radio report about an intriguing experiment by the University of New Hampshire football team caught my attention.[4] Erik Swartz, a professor of kinesiology at the university, hypothesized that concussions could be reduced if players became more actively aware of their tackling technique by not wearing helmets. He divided the team up into two 25-player squads for research purposes. One group did tackling drills without helmets, while the other ran the same drills wearing helmets. The players without helmets were encouraged to keep their heads up while tackling, using their torsos for chest-to-chest point-of-contact tackling. The idea was to see if they would learn safer form, using their arms and shoulders during tackles, thereby better protecting the brain from impact forces. Swartz measured the force delivered to the head in both groups of players, through a sensor placed behind the ear. This was just the first phase of his study, and at that time he was hoping to collect more data from high school teams.

"If you look on the sidelines, let's say, after there's a touchdown in football, oftentimes the players will head-butt . . . to celebrate," Swartz says in the NPR story. "They probably wouldn't do that if they didn't have a helmet on."

It's an interesting idea, one certainly worthy of more research.

MOUTHGUARDS

Many athletes across the spectrum of sports wear mouthguards during play. Some do so just to follow the rules, others for their obvious protective attributes. The primary role of a mouth-guard is to protect the teeth, gums, jaw, or chin from breakage or other damage due to blows and forces received during play. Think about what happens with elbows during rebounding scrums or about a shoulder that thrusts up into the jaw while a player is going for a soccer ball. In both cases, forces, especially ones directed upward, can strike hard into the mouth, chin and jaw.

Wearing a mouthguard can also help protect the brain in contact situations, by muting the transmission of force through the skull, lower jaw, and teeth. Some mouthguard manufac-turers, however, claim that mouthguards can help minimize concussive forces delivered to any area of the head. To date, there is not enough science to back this claim. So as a general rule, I tell my patients that mouthguards are essential in con-tact sports for oral protection and that they may provide some small level of increased protection against concussion in a mi-nority of impacts.

Like helmets, mouthguards should be appropriate to the sport, with the proper fit and maintenance. Fit-it-yourself mouthguards, the cheapest option, are available at drugstores and sporting goods stores. The fitting process is simple: The bite tray is boiled to soften the plastic and then fit to the mouth by having the player bite down on it for a few mo-ments while it is cooling and setting. The player's unique bite imprint is then permanently etched into the thermoplas-tic form. The main issue with fit-it-yourself mouthguards is that they are not as durable or as thick as professionally made custom ones. A thicker material provides a better layer of protection in the mouth.

A custom-fitted mouthguard can be constructed by your family dentist or a specialty sport equipment company. Custom mouthguards are made of acrylic and have a laminating film to make them more durable. They also can be made with colors or team logos for some fashion flair.

No matter what type of mouthguard you choose, it's good to follow a few practices to maintain their integrity: Don't chew on them, don't take them out and jam them into facemasks, clean them regularly, and try not to expose them to extreme heat or cold (for example, by leaving them in a car). A bent, torn, or warped mouthguard is not effective. As children grow, they will periodically need new mouthguards. Youth athletes who have orthodontic devices like braces or expanders should check with their orthodontists about how to best protect their mouths during sports.

IMPACT SENSORS

Wearable technology has become mainstream in the fitness world with items like the Fitbit, the Jawbone, or even the multifunctional Apple Watch. This kind of technology has also made its way onto the sports concussion scene. Impact sensors, which are small devices placed in helmets, headbands, or mouthguards or worn directly on the skin, provide estimates of the frequency, locations, and amounts of force an athlete's brain incurs during games or practices. The collection of data from these sensors is a valuable tool for scientific and medical researchers trying to reach evidence-based conclusions about what happens to the body and brain during competition.

It's important to realize, however, that impact sensors provide only an estimate of what the brain actually experiences. Each type of sensor has its own limitations. Their use is still developing as the technology advances and our experience with them grows.

One of the holy grails of the concussion world, of course, is a test or technology that would provide a real-time indication that somebody has been injured. Some manufacturers of commercially available impact sensors make scientifically unsubstantiated claims that by monitoring forces, their products can provide that red light/green light concussion sign.

Still, even if they cannot provide anything close to diagnostic certainty, impact sensors can serve an important function by making responsible medical personnel aware of potential concussions. These devices typically are designed to link up through Bluetooth to a smart phone or computer, giving researchers, medical personnel, or parents a real-time assessment of how many hits an athlete has taken, and with how much force. When a predetermined threshold is exceeded, medical personnel can then call the player off the field for a concussion evaluation. Newer devices even integrate a GPS component that sends a locator signal for help if an athlete breaks the threshold for a concussive blow while doing a solo activity such as skiing or mountain biking.

But if every concussion is unique, and different levels of force affect each athlete differently, how can a single sensor make an individualized and contextualized determination of trouble? A slight blow, something that may not register as serious enough to cause a concussion, can happen during a game and cause brain trauma. And a big hit, forceful enough to set the sensor off, could result in no injury.

The answer is that a sensor is simply a piece of technology that collects data. We still need to have athletic trainers, qualified medical staff, and informed parents and coaches involved in assessing and helping potentially injured athletes.

Our technology-driven culture loves to transform things into apps. We can order a pizza from the shop around the corner, shoes from another country, or even a car from another state via a smartphone. We can also track our heart rate, calories consumed, and steps taken. But we cannot—yet—rely on a sensor to accurately let us know when a concussive event has occurred. There is a danger in buying into impact sensors as a magical safety switch to tell us whether or a concussion has happened. Knowing statistics on every hit a player took on a football field isn't useful unless that knowledge is interpreted thoughtfully and in context.

SIMPLE THINGS: STRENGTH
AND HYDRATION

Sometimes the simplest things are the most powerful. We are starting to understand more about the role of neck strength in preventing concussion and long-term brain injury. Studies have shown there is an anatomical difference in neck strength between male and female athletes, one that is significant enough that it may be a factor in why girls and women sustain concussions more easily. Less neck strength means less ability to absorb rotational or linear forces, which makes the brain more vulnerable to being jarred by whiplash and other kinds of injury.

For increased protection against concussion, especially in female athletes, I recommend carefully considering neck strengthening and seeking guidance from a trained strength professional on proper neck alignment. Strength and conditioning experts can develop age- and sport-appropriate exercises to help strengthen the neck, and coaches can keep a sharp eye on technique to ensure proper form.

One of the risk factors for brain injury that is given the least thought is poor hydration. Being dehydrated during play can cause a lot of things: cramping, poor performance, and overall discomfort. But if the hydration deficit is severe enough, it may also cause a decrease in cerebrospinal fluid, which the brain relies on for cushioning during impact. Let's use another egg analogy. Now the shell is the skull, the yolk is the brain, and the cerebrospinal fluid is the egg white. When the egg is shaken, the white protects the yolk from crashing into the shell. So not hydrating properly can leave the brain a bit more vulnerable during impact. Not only that, but since athletic performance usually drops when an athlete is dehydrated, it stands to reason that technique also worsens and the chances of having an accident increase.

The other effect that dehydration might have is on symptom production. If a person is even mildly dehydrated, the brain may more easily produce symptoms. If the dehydration is bad enough, sometimes symptoms that look just like concussion occur, further clouding the picture of an already difficult diagnostic puzzle.

Thankfully, stories of coaches withholding fluids during practice as a punishment or performance inducement are quickly fading away as the dangers of dehydration become better known. Hydration is a critical facet of athletic health and performance and must be monitored. My experience tells me, for example, that if care isn't taken, injury rates tend to be higher during the second practice of two-practice-a-day training camps. Why? Most likely because athletes' technique may worsen a little—or even a lot—when they are more tired and dehydrated. These are clear factors that can make the difference between getting hurt and staying healthy. Making sure athletes get enough fluid for the weather and their exertion level can go a long way toward keeping their brains safer and their performance levels strong.

TECHNIQUE AS PROTECTION

Using proper techniques for tackling, heading, checking, and other important athletic maneuvers also can help an athlete have a successful and safe career. A lot of thought is now going into ways of teaching sports techniques, how athletes interpret and enact those lessons, and the effects these efforts may have on concussion rates. National groups such as USA Football and USA Hockey are making efforts to educate parents, coaches, and athletes across the population about ways that technique can make those sports safer. The biggest challenge is often at the beginner levels of sports, where coaches tend to be parent volunteers who may rely on the outdated techniques and methods by which they learned the sport. Staying current with technique, actively reviewing it during practices, and keeping a watchful eye on how athletes are executing maneuvers during games can be excellent ways to build a better, safer game.

Improving how players tackle, with a focus on reducing forces to the head, could be a big step forward for football. Some coaches, however, argue that their teams will not be as effective—or successful—if they radically change technique from the tried and true. The experience of the Seattle Seahawks might convince them otherwise.

Seahawks head coach Pete Carroll is at the top of his profession as one of only three coaches to win both the Super

Bowl and a college football championship. Carroll's teams are known for playing smart, disciplined football with some offensive flair. They also play using Carroll's modified tackling technique, which he calls *Hawk tackling*. This technique is designed to take the head and helmet out of tackling and reduce injuries. It may sound a little crazy that a top-tier NFL coach is trying to teach a less aggressive tackling technique, but Carroll really believes, and his record supports the idea, that taking the head out of tackling is not a barrier to winning football games.

Carroll teaches tackling as something done from the shoulders down, with a focus on wrapping the arms up around the waist and avoiding leading or finishing with the helmet. He made a video in 2014 to explain his tackling approach and sent it to 14,000 high school football teams and 8,000 youth programs, hoping to get them all to reconsider their techniques in order to better protect the heads of their young players.

"There's so much talk around the league and around the game of football right now that I wanted to see if we could contribute to helping people understand how you could play this game and do it in a great fashion and continue to promote the game," Carroll said about his rethinking of techniques.[5] "This is a concept we've been working on for a long time and something that's built into our makeup. But we just thought it would be worth sharing, and really hoping that it works its way through high school football and youth football to teach kids at an early age how to tackle and how to take care of themselves and play this game really fast and hard in absolutely the safest way possible."

I like that Carroll is trying to improve how football is played not only at the highest level of football but at all levels. Starting off with safer technique can make all the difference for an athlete. Even the youngest athletes need to be watched for technique. If you think that tiny football players can't hurt themselves if they ram their heads together while goofing around during practice, you're mistaken. And of course, youth coaches need to be up on the best practices for tackling to help teach and enforce them.

In sports with aerial elements, such as cheerleading, skating, gymnastics, skiing, snowboarding, and diving, it's essential to have a solid foundation in the basics before trying more difficult moves. At the highest levels, the best athletes practice drilling the most complicated maneuvers in safe settings before "going live." Youth athletics can follow their example by using proper floor padding and safety equipment, having athletes do a few extra run-throughs on the harness, and having coaches keep a watchful eye on technique. These practices will help young athletes stay safe while advancing their performance.

US soccer star Kate Markgraf (Chapters 7 and 8) thinks soccer could be made safer through an emphasis on better heading techniques. She also knows about the measurable difference in neck strength between males and females and understands that female soccer players may have higher concussion rates than males. She thinks the women's game could be improved through detailed study of neck strength and, if warranted, a focus on appropriate neck strengthening.

"My nonscientific thought is, headers could be made safer if players consistently did them the right way, had the proper techniques," Markgraf says. "It's on the coaches to teach that, on the players to then execute it. Headers have place in the game, if they are done correctly."

FOLLOWING THE RULES

If you went online and searched for the rulebooks for the NBA, NFL, pro soccer, or any other popular organized sport, you would find that each one has hundreds of regulations, covering every aspect of the game from timeouts and illegal plays to the dimensions of the playing surface, the equipment used, and player rosters. Many of the rules are in place to protect player health and safety. Some of those rules have been around for decades or more, but many are new and represent significant changes designed to improve safety.

Major League Baseball changed its rules for the 2014 season, increasing protection for players by banning collisions at the plate unless the catcher has the ball or is fielding a throw. Violent collisions at the plate have a long history in baseball, but the sport recognized the damage—namely, concussions in catchers—that was resulting from the play.

Rules are useless, however, unless they are consistently and correctly enforced. Athletes come into my office with concussions that they say stemmed from a dirty play or a situation that an official did not enforce correctly.

Officiating sports is not easy, however. It requires training, skill, practice, and a whole lot of thick skin. Officials at every level are expected to call a good game, keep it safe, and keep it fair. But nobody wants to compete in, let alone watch, a game that is dominated by officials calling every little thing. Some discretion is always smart, and the best officials at any level know when to let players play and when to step in. It can definitely be a rough job. Pressures come from players, coaches, fans, and, in youth sports, very vocal parents. For all of these reasons, I have the utmost respect for our sports officials and the job they do.

And with increased concern about concussion, we are asking more of them than ever before. Officials are now given very specific responsibilities regarding looking out for signs of brain trauma in athletes.

Having coaches, officials, and players keep up on the rules, and then having the rules actively and consistently enforced, can lead to a safer game. Overly aggressive play can lead to injury, as can cheap shots. There is so much about the run of play that cannot be controlled, but intelligent enforcement of existing rules—at all levels of sports—can go a long way to creating a better atmosphere for athletes.

Coaches who promote bending the rules or being overly aggressive do not serve the best interests of their athletes or their sport. The same goes for players with a dirty or overly aggressive approach to play. For the good of everyone, they need to be re-educated to play at a safer level or be banned from their sport.

BASELINE TESTING

Like impact sensors, baseline testing is a potentially useful method for collecting data that may provide some benefit in clinical decision-making. If done correctly, it can provide a snapshot in time of brain function. Baseline testing, as discussed earlier, works well as a type of neurological metric that can be used for comparison during a post-injury situation and become part of a comprehensive decision-making process.

As baseline testing becomes more widespread, thanks to now popular mandates from school districts and leagues, more and more products are flooding the market, with some overzealous companies and medical professionals touting that their tests provide ways to protect athletes from injury or diagnose concussion. You will continue to hear about this or that test, or some other new technology, that somebody says will "make the difference" and allow medical personnel, or even coaches or parents, to diagnose concussion on the sideline.

Beware of these claims! These tests do not diagnose concussion and doing baseline testing is not like taking out an insurance policy against concussion or brain trauma. Remember, baseline testing of any sort works best when administered by qualified medical professionals and when interpreted and used correctly as part of the recovery process if a concussion has indeed occurred.

OFF THE BEATEN PATH

There is rarely one solution to a complex medical issue. Patients can opt for traditional medicine, experimental treatments, holistic or natural approaches, and, sadly, "cures" that are based on less-than-scrupulous practices.

Researchers are looking at many ways to try to heal the brain after trauma, and before anyone jumps into a "miracle" concussion cure, rigorous testing and proof are needed. I have had many patients who have tried specific diets, vitamins, or supplements to fix post-concussion symptoms, and sometimes they do improve. But you can't just go to the health food store and buy various pills to "fix" a concussion itself. While I believe in the overall role of vitamins and supplements in health if used correctly, I advise my patients to think carefully about using them and to ask the advice of a physician. An example of a supplement I do often find useful is melatonin, which I frequently tell patients who have sleep issues to try.

Eating right and getting proper rest are huge assets to getting well, as is exercising. Again, integrating a qualified medical professional into the assessment and discussion of treatment can lead to options that are holistic.

For example, you may hear commercials claiming that treatments such as hyperbaric chamber therapy can heal concussions. That treatment doesn't work any better than using pressurized oxygen, according to a randomized clinical trial on US military members with post-concussive issues whose results appeared in the January 2015 issue of *JAMA Internal Medicine*.[6] And yet the claims are still being made, and many people are paying thousands of dollars for hyperbaric treatment in the hope of improvement.

I've also heard about alternative medical treatments that use flashing-light therapy to "reorient" the brain, fringe or unusual types of "brain scans," and gyroscopes that spin and flip athletes around like they are training to be astronauts—all to help with post-concussive issues. A November 2013 article in *The New Republic* wonders openly if concussion treatments have entered a "snake-oil phase."[7]

Bottom line, you need to be careful and cautious regardless of what type of treatment, protective equipment, or technology you're considering. It's OK to be a little cynical and look out for people or organizations that are trying to make a buck or two taking advantage of fear and worry about the concussion "crisis."

REFERENCES

1. Stamp J. Leatherhead to radio-head: the evolution of the football helmet. October 1, 2012. http://www.smithsonianmag.com/arts-culture/leatherhead-to-radio-head-the-evolution-of-the-football-helmet-56585562/?no-ist.

2. Rose B. Olympic snowboarder splits helmet in violent slopestyle crash. February 9, 2014. http://www.si.com/extra-mustard/2014/02/09/olympic-snowboarder-splits-helmet-in-violent-slopestyle-crash.

3. Virginia Tech helmet ratings. Translating research to reduce concussion risk. http://www.beam.vt.edu/helmet/index.php.

4. Rodolico J. Football players drill without helmets to curb concussions. December 11, 2014. http://www.npr.org/blogs/health/2014/12/11/370116343/solving-football-s-concussion-problem-practice-without-helmets.

5. Farnsworth C. Pete Carroll tackles a serious issue with instructional video. July 28, 2014. http://www.seahawks.com/news/2014/07/28/pete-carroll-tackles-serious-issue-instructional-video.

6. Miller RS, Weaver LK, Bahraini N, et al. Effects of hyperbaric oxygen on symptoms and quality of life among service members with persistent postconcussion symptoms: a randomized clinical trial. *JAMA Internal Medicine* 2015 Jan;175(1):43–52. doi: 10.1001/jamainternmed.2014.5479.

7. Schwartz J. These fringe doctors say they can cure NFL concussion victims. *The New Republic.* November 17, 2013. http://www.newrepublic.com/article/115527/nfl-concussion-crisis-doctors-use-alternative-medicine.

TEN

CONTROLLING THE MESSAGING
OF CONCUSSION

In a classic moment from American cinema, the character Maxwell Scott, a newspaper editor in the Western tale *The Man Who Shot Liberty Valance* (1962), is asked if he is going to use recently confirmed facts to correct the public's understanding of the details of a well-known murder. The truth, it seems, tells a story much different from, and much less compelling than, the currently accepted version.

Scott throws his notebook in the fire and says: "No, sir. This is the West, sir. When the legend becomes fact, print the legend."

I love that movie, always have. John Wayne and Jimmy Stewart at their finest!

One of its many powerful themes that still holds true today is how the media controls public perception, and how that perception, if left unchallenged, can replace reality in people's minds. This isn't a novel idea, of course. Any observer or student of the media comes to understand the power that lies in strong and consistent messaging. Strong messages and compelling stories sold newspapers back in the "yellow journalism" era of the 1900s. They continue to do so in our digital-based age, even if business success in now measured not by newsstand sales but by the cold metrics of Internet clicks, social media hits, and virality. Even as the media have fractured into pieces, splintering from newspapers, television and radio into Twitter, Facebook, texting, YouTube, and much more, the influence of messaging remains the same whenever an important issue of the day captures the public's attention. The multitudes of voices speaking about concussion in sports across media formats, whether it is a sports fan with no medical knowledge on Twitter, a former NFL player doing color commentary on ESPN, a writer with *Sports Illustrated*, or even a TMZ tabloid reporter, all lend to the confusing cacophony. But the idea is always the same: driving traffic, gaining a following, and, if a business is involved, making money. It's a very powerful part of our global society.

GETTING CONCUSSION RISK WRONG

In the fall of 2009, I discovered firsthand the media's power in controlling messages about concussions in sports. I was walking through the University of Michigan's hospital, on my way to give grand rounds (the medical school practice of presenting particular cases and topics to students and other doctors) to the Department of Neurology. The chair of my department stopped me in the hallway, asking if I had seen the front page of that morning's *New York Times*. I hadn't, so he went to pick one up for me, promising that it was relevant to my upcoming talk.

The topic of my lecture that morning was the need for neurology to get deeply involved in sports concussion and to commit to improving the neurological care of athletes at all levels. Even in 2009, I had seen too often the oversimplification in the media of the issues surrounding sports concussion. "Experts" of all types, but few physicians and even fewer neurologists, had begun speaking out to question the safety of sports, especially American football. Given what the field of neurology represents, I felt strongly that it had to get involved and partner with other medical specialties to help keep the conversation constructive, strongly rooted in science, and, most importantly, helpful for our patients.

When my department chair handed me the paper, just a few moments before I was to speak, I was greeted with a most intriguing front-page headline. It certainly was one that I would have never expected to see in one of the world's largest and most influential mainstream newspapers: "Dementia Risk Seen in Players in N.F.L. Study."[1]

Wow. That was a serious headline. All the time and effort I and my colleagues had invested in educating our patients and the public, doing research, and providing care seemed to paying off. To see that story in the *New York Times* was a game changer. Finally! People were starting to pay attention.

There was only one problem.

To my mind, that headline could mean only that a group of researchers must have conducted some groundbreaking research and published a substantial epidemiological study on NFL players. I was particularly intrigued because that would mean that I wasn't aware of some very important ongoing research on athletes and neurology. The potential existence of a new group of colleagues to interact with, to share ideas and data with, was always exciting, especially back then, when very few medical researchers were spending significant time on these issues.

The word "risk" in the headline caught my attention the most. This term is used in conversations about medical conditions all the time. To a physician or scientist, however, the term is not used lightly and has a very specific meaning. A series of conditions must be met before we agree that some factor is a risk for developing a medical condition, the most important of these being a significant amount of reproducible evidence. Part of the evidence must speak to a certain statistical relationship: The exposure in question should be established to be present to a greater extent than we would expect to see by chance alone in the population affected by the condition being discussed (where by "population" we mean the population as a whole, not just a collection of individuals). There must also be an underpinning of basic science principles, such as how the factor might cause the condition at a cellular level.

When I was finished with my lecture and had a few moments to read the story carefully, however, I learned that the study in question was a phone survey—hardly the type of research that should ever be used to describe a medical risk. Because the study was designed to describe the overall physical, mental, and social health of former NFL players, respondents were asked many questions, spanning a variety of topics. Only one question had to do with dementing illness: Former players were asked whether or not they had a diagnosis of dementia or had complained to a doctor about their memory. The players were asked for no further details, and the researchers sought no independent confirmation of their responses.

The NFL had commissioned the study, and it was not peer-reviewed or published in the medical literature. As the story "grew legs" in the weeks that followed, the fact that the NFL had sponsored the study was stated numerous times across the media. No story, however, took the time or space to provide even a reasonably complete or accurate version of the facts. Repeated over and over, a new "truth" was established: that playing football caused dementia. There was very little if any attention paid to how often this might be the case or how established the relationship really was. It just "was."

Nonetheless that headline and the conversation it started went on to define the sports concussion landscape. The effects can still be felt today. Playing in the NFL is now widely assumed to be an established risk factor for dementia. The problem is that a memorable headline or grabbing the public's attention doesn't come from a measured, complete, and fair description of what we know right now about sports-related brain trauma as a risk for dementia.

CONCUSSION IN THE POLITICAL THEATER

Just like in the media, oversimplification for the purpose of messaging often shows up in our political process.

In 2010, I had the honor of being asked to provide testimony for a US House of Representatives Judiciary Committee hearing on legal issues relating to football head injuries. I was asked to present to the hearing because of my unique role as a neurologist who was also a team physician for an NCAA Division I athletic program, working at the University of Michigan. I spent several days preparing my testimony. I wanted to present a thoughtful take on the issues before the committee, drawing on my experience and training and highlighting the matters I felt were critically important for my patients.

Before it was my turn, the committee took the testimony of Dr. Ira Casson, a physician who conducted research on concussion and other brain trauma for the NFL. When he was finished, Dr. Casson fielded many questions from the members of Congress conducting the hearing. What was fascinating to me was that it didn't matter much what questions they asked or how he answered, because the overall narrative was already established and quite clear: Dr. Casson was absolutely certain there was no connection between playing in the NFL and having a brain disease later in life.

Did he actually say that? No, he didn't. Even so, one member of Congress took this narrative so far as to start referring to Dr. Casson as "Dr. No."

The Judiciary Committee also heard from Dr. Bennet Omalu, a neuropathologist who helped describe the earliest cases of CTE in deceased NFL players, and someone who clearly thought that the chronic exposure to football impacts was the connecting link. (He is now more famous as the basis for the main character in the 2015 movie *Concussion*, where he was portrayed by Will Smith.) Dr. Omalu gave very passionate testimony to the committee, describing this newly discovered relationship and the need for swift and significant action. By the time he was finished, the narrative had solidified around a classic good-versus-evil plot, as Dr. Omalu was then referred to as "Dr. Yes." He was then asked questions that helped support his testimony, further defining his position on the side of good and as the clear and complete opposite of "Dr. No."

When it was my turn, I didn't make any dramatic claims, one way or the other, regarding the popular take on concussion. I spoke as a physician and scientist with an opinion based on established science, giving significant deference to what we don't know, which was then (and still is) far more than what we do know. After my "non-controversial" testimony, I was asked only one question: "Was there was anything that Dr. Casson said that you agreed with?"

I sat there a little stunned. I didn't expect these proceedings to allow for a detailed discussion of science. Indeed, I went into that room knowing that the hearing would be more about telling a story that would turn heads, collect clicks, and further define public opinion. Still, it was a bit shocking to be so blatantly pulled in to the fray.

I took a moment, and a breath, and answered. What struck me about the testimony of "Dr. No" and "Dr. Yes," I offered, was that the two actually had a good bit in common if you considered only the facts they stated, without all of the emotional language. In the end, both were supportive of the concept that repetitive brain trauma could be a risk factor for a neurological disease, and both felt that we needed to know more. So when I had collected my thoughts and made the point that the perceived gap between the two sides (a simple ballot, if you will: Vote Yes! or Vote No!) had little to do with what their scientific opinions were and more to do with how they were speaking and how they were being portrayed, I braced for consequences of my honesty. Surely, the committee wouldn't let me get away with not taking a side.

I'll never forget the awkward, but thankfully brief, silence when I was done speaking, as well as the momentary blank looks from the committee members. They were trying to find a way to translate my words into something that would fit their narrative. They wanted to put me on one side or the other. When they couldn't, they moved on. I didn't field another question the rest of the afternoon.

I left the hearing a little bit irritated, and certainly disappointed, by the theater it represented and the opportunity that had been missed. What I said that day is still true today. There is enough scientific evidence for us to be concerned about a causal relationship between sports-related contact and CTE or other long-term brain health issues. At the same time, there is not nearly enough evidence for us to say that we understand that relationship.

Let's face it: Whether in the media or in the political process, medical science typically does not make for good storytelling. I have a completely unrealistic fantasy that someday there will be *Researching With the Stars* or a non–soap opera look at medical science on TV. Wouldn't it be fascinating if there were! But yes, probably too boring for popular consumption. Ryan Seacrest probably would not be interested in hosting that show.

For any medical or scientific issue to significantly capture the public's attention, it seems, a highly charged and emotional narrative must be attached to it. At least I'm afraid that's what we have in the case of sports and brain trauma. Over the past five or six years, the public has been hearing from those individuals who have the loudest megaphones and get in front of the most cameras. People who are passionate about athletes and concussions but have little scientific knowledge or training have taken to mass and social media in force to put out their own personal conclusions—mostly without being challenged. The people who get the most influential opportunities to be heard, to no one's surprise, are most often those with the most dramatic and impassioned messages, whether their messages are based on facts or not.

So, as the fictional Mr. Scott in that classic 1962 Western noted, when legend becomes fact, you go with the legend. Unfortunately, in this case, lives are being affected negatively every single day because critical thought takes a back seat while emotional narratives play the starring role.

But I am not ready to throw my notebook into the fireplace.

THE MEDIA AS A SOURCE FOR MEDICAL INFORMATION

I often find myself giving out the general advice "Get your medical information from medical experts, not media ones." I do this in large part because of what I described above, the media's need to tell a compelling story. The other reason is that communicating clearly about complex medical issues can be very difficult. Finding concise yet accurate ways to do these issues justice can be nearly impossible, especially when one is trying to communicate within the user-driven social media venues of Twitter or Facebook.

Observing media professionals as they discuss athletes' brain health, it's disturbing to find that the word *concussion* is used more often incorrectly than correctly. Most often I see or hear it used as a catch-all term for trauma-related brain health issues in athletes. Concussion is a very common injury that occurs not only in sports but also as the result of ordinary life activities. When the public perceptions of concussion shifted from a potentially serious but transient injury to one that was always serious and could potentially change your life forever, medical professionals started to see a dramatic change in behavior. Now, for example, it's not uncommon that a patient will come to my clinic wondering if one, quite typical concussion they experienced decades ago could still be causing headaches or memory difficulties. Even more concerning are the many patients who are convinced they are just biding time until dementia sets in because they played a contact sport in high school. The troubling "concussion = dementia" narrative has gained traction from anecdotal reports spread in the media without any context.

Other common communication missteps center around how concussion is diagnosed. When you listen to commentators covering sporting events you could easily come away with the idea that concussion diagnosis and management is simply a matter of following protocols. If the steps are outlined in enough detail and followed to a T, then diagnosis should be easy, goes the thinking. While there is definitely an important role for protocols in concussion diagnosis and management, when protocols take the place of thinking, patients suffer.

So whenever you come across the words "concussion protocol," be a little cautious. Look carefully for evidence that the protocol in question has been put in place for the wrong reasons. Often protocols are designed to provide legal protection for sports teams or institutions rather than for the benefit of athlete health and safety. Other times, protocols are nothing more than administrative hoops to jump through or medical shortcuts to make up for a lack of resources. In the end, any protocol is only as good as the medical professionals, coaches, and administrators responsible for carrying it out.

I cannot emphasize this concept enough. The difference between adhering strictly and exclusively to protocols and providing proper medical care is like the difference between always following a recipe to the letter, with the exact same ingredients, so that you end up with exactly the same dinner entrée, and going to the farmer's market, seeing what items you have to work with, and then having the skill and experience to put them together in a way that produces something desirable. Much like what's available at the local farmer's market, the available facts and conditions will be different for every concussion. And just as cooking requires a particular set of skills, many particular neurological skills are required to manage concussions. There is no one recipe to manage them all.

Whatever the particular messaging about concussion is, I have come to realize over the years that in most cases, journalists do want to get the information right. However, they cannot be right all the time, and just because something is in print or broadcast, that doesn't make it the truth. I understand that it can be hard to know from the outside looking in what is correct and what isn't. My best advice is to take everything in the media with a little grain of salt.

I don't want to be too critical of the media, however. I've definitely come to appreciate the institution of journalism for the incredibly important role it plays. And I have tremendous respect as well for those individual journalists who question the assumptions, dig a little harder to understand the more difficult concepts, and then manage to turn around and craft a clear and nuanced message for public consumption.

POPULAR CULTURE
AND YOUTH SPORTS

It can be very informative and helpful to take a look back and try to understand how pop culture, especially movies and TV, may have influenced the thinking of parents of youth athletes over the years. We did not just arrive at today's notion of athletics as a test of character and strength. American culture is not unique in celebrating athletes as warriors. The Roman gladiators set the standard for the narrative of competing through pain and being celebrated for victory while overcoming serious injury. Ancient audiences packed arenas to watch spectacles of hand-to-hand, and sometimes man-versus-animal, athletic combat.[2]

The Olympic movement, both ancient and modern, centers on the concept of athletes' enduring challenges, sometimes painful or risky, as a price for final victory. Marathoners, for example, will feel the painful burn of their muscles being depleted during their long run, but they keep going. Boxers are bloodied but keep fighting to score points or a knockout. Those competitors who push through pain to win are rewarded with medals and acclaim. More recently, female athletes have been added to the ranks of warrior athletes, a sign of our society's including all who compete within the philosophy that pain, injury, and even permanent physical damage should be risked for victory.

The list of movies that celebrate the warrior athlete who overcomes injury is long. The "Rocky" series finds Sylvester Stallone's title character frequently bleeding and punished before he wins. The 1974 football movie *The Longest Yard* shows Burt Reynolds playing through a serious knee injury. The 2004 movie *Million Dollar Baby* has Hilary Swank's character, Maggie, tragically break her neck in the boxing ring during a title fight. Even in the 1992 comedy *A League of Their Own*, Tom Hanks memorably utters the catchphrase "There's no crying in baseball" to decry weakness in the Rockford Peaches (and, by implication, sports in general). And these are just a few of the most memorable characters and scenes in the American sports movie canon in the past 40 years. Many, many more have left their mark in significant ways on our understanding of the importance to athletics of stoically enduring injury.

The warrior-athlete mentality is reinforced not just by scripted entertainment but by live sporting events and the "legends" they give rise to. NFL Films and ESPN once curated dramatic montages, set to pulse-pounding orchestral music, of "big hits" in football, showing off the violence and raw strength of the game. Hockey fight compilations from the 1980s and 1990s, especially ones featuring "enforcers" Tie Domi, Stu Grimson, or the late Bob Probert, still find thousands of viewers on YouTube. Crowds still jump to their feet in excitement when fights (now less common) break out in professional hockey.

And we could go on and on about the athletes who are remembered and revered for playing at their best, or sometimes less than best, through obvious injury. Being an athlete, especially at the elite levels, frequently demands being able to go through pain and keep competing.

US gymnast Kerri Strug memorably completed a vault in which she essentially landed on one foot because of a badly sprained left ankle to help clinch the team gold medal at the 1996 Atlanta Olympics. Champion diver Greg Louganis hit the board during the 1988 Seoul Olympics, gashing the back of his head and needing five stitches, but kept competing and won the gold.[3] Toronto Maple Leafs defenseman Bobby Baun had his right leg broken by a Gordie Howe slap shot late in the third period of a game, was carried off the ice on a stretcher, received painkillers, and returned to score the game-winning goal in overtime during the 1964 Stanley Cup finals.[4]

Live and TV audiences watched the sock of Red Sox pitcher Curt Schilling turn red from blood oozing from a fresh surgical incision as he threw seven innings of winning baseball against the Yankees at Yankee Stadium during Game 6 of the

2004 American League Championship Series.[5] And in one of the still most discussed performances in professional soccer, goalie Bert Trautmann played through a broken neck—yes, according to media reports, a visibly broken neck—to help Manchester City win 3–1 over Birmingham City and capture the 1956 FA Cup. Trautmann returned to the pitch after a serious collision with an opponent while trying to score. He not only broke his neck, but was also knocked unconscious.[6]

In light of this powerful imagery, and considering that concussions are not visibly obvious—not nearly as clear as a boxer's being knocked cold in the ring by a savage left hook or a goalie's lying still on the pitch from a collision—how do we reconcile wanting our children to be disciplined and "tough" athletes with protecting their brain health? How do we take concussion seriously without completely losing positive values of sports like overcoming adversity, sportsmanship, working as a collective, being disciplined, and respecting coaches and officials?

PRESERVING SPORTS WHILE PROTECTING BRAINS

What is best way to put into perspective the sporting moments, memories, and cultural touchstones that may influence our thinking on concussions and how to be an athlete?

One thing we must do is be honest about the ways the mass media, the Internet, and social media, as well as our peers, have shaped our feelings about concussions and sports. The things everyone used to celebrate, such as a quarterback's getting "destroyed" by a charging linebacker, are now viewed by many as cringeworthy and as representing what's wrong with football.

Andrei Markovits, a professor of political sciences and sociology at the University of Michigan, is an expert analyst on global sporting culture and on how sociology and politics intermingle with athletics. He is also a big sports fan who has been watching the evolving discourse on concussions in sports. Markovits sees the change in North America from viewing concussions as nothing much to worry about to seeing them as a serious concern as rooted in a larger societal context.

"It comes back to three things: We have become a more empathetic, compassionate society since the late-1960s, [so] we are [more] inclined to protect our children; the rise of the women's movement, as women have more financial and political power, which gives women the power to change public discourse in the world; and finally, we are more health-conscious overall," says Markovits. "The moms have more say, and they do not want their children to get hurt. They see football as leading to concussions, so they will put their foot down and say they do not want their child playing football. We are in a more protective world, a more feminine world, which are not bad things. We are more compassionate and careful about risks, but that also will lead to being reactionary about perceived dangers such as concussions."

I am frequently asked where I see sports going in the future in light of the concerns over athletes' brain health. Will there be football as we know it? Should hockey allow checking? Should we remove all contact from sports? Maybe rugby really is safer than American tackle football? Would I let my son play football?

Trying to accept the aggression and violence in our sports, which are sometimes intrinsic to the sport itself, is challenging. Football, at its most basic level, cannot be played without players' tackling or running into each other, which will cause injuries. Auto racing, especially on high-speed oval courses, will have crashes, sometimes leaving drivers permanently injured or even dead. Divers will always aim to land head first into the pool and will sometimes, like Louganis, accidentally smack their heads on the board.

The reality is, we cannot take all the risk out of sports. In many ways we understand that minimizing risk should be a priority, but in the end, risk is all around us every day, whether we play sports or not. By exposing ourselves to some to the intrinsic health risks of playing sports, we are also opening ourselves up to incredible opportunities for personal growth and accomplishment. Keeping this equation in mind, understanding both the risks and the benefits of sport is essential to individual and societal growth.

All of us in sports, from medical staff to coaches to leagues and players, seek to find ways to move our games into realms of improved safety without taking away their spirit. Football, at all levels, has made rule changes to eliminate injury-causing tackles like chop blocks and to protect quarterbacks and kickers from being unnecessarily roughed up.

Sports are man-made in every way. The rules are flexible and arbitrary. As a society, we can work to move our sports in the direction of protecting our athletes from unnecessary harm. But we cannot eliminate all elements of danger. The random occurrences, and our responses to those unexpected events play after play, are the human elements that we emotionally connect to. If we knew the outcome of every play, every last-second free throw, every championship game, or every putt, why would we participate in or watch sports?

RISK VERSUS BENEFIT: PUTTING IT ALL TOGETHER

I've talked a lot about many of the benefits of sports, as well as some of the potential harms. As a neurologist, I've dedicated my professional life to improving the neurological health of athletes at all levels of play. When I began that quest, it was a very natural thing to focus on the potential dangers and to work to minimize risk and improve outcome after injury. I thought a lot about my own childhood playing ice hockey in

Michigan. I thought about the concussions I myself had had, about my kids and what sports they might play, and about the injuries they could get.

If you had asked me in the beginning of my career, I would have said that improving the neurological health of athletes meant mainly protecting them from injury and treating them with the best possible medical care when they were hurt.

What I came to appreciate later were the real negative health effects that can come from not playing sports. As my appreciation for this side of the risk–benefit balance grew, I began to see a larger picture. Every person has his or her own set of traits that add up to a uniquely individual relationship with sports. Sure, you can put people into groups: the recreational athletes, the "serious" ones, and the elite or professional players. You can group sports into different risk profiles too: collision, contact, or non-contact. But you also have to consider different personalities, psychologies, and ways of thinking.

One thing is clear: Critical thought and a comprehensive approach to medical care are the keys to maximizing brain health over a lifetime. Time and time again, I see people making decisions about participation in sports too quickly, with too many assumptions, and with too many variables left unaccounted for. Our kids, our athletes, all of us, deserve better.

It's a shared responsibility, but one I think we can all live with.

In sports, it's called teamwork.

REFERENCES

1. Schwarz A. Dementia risk seen in players in N.F.L. study. *New York Times.* September 29, 2009. http://www.nytimes.com/2009/09/30/sports/football/30dementia.html.

2. Andrews E. 10 things you may not know about Roman gladiators. March 4, 2014. http://www.history.com/news/history-lists/10-things-you-may-not-know-about-roman-gladiators.

3. Plaschke B. Greg Louganis remembers the Olympic dive that made history. *Los Angeles Times.* September 12, 2013. http://articles.latimes.com/2013/sep/12/sports/la-sp-plaschke-louganis-20130913.

4. Hunter P. 50 years later, Maple Leafs legend Bobby Baun still unstoppable. *Toronto Star.* April 11, 2014. http://www.thestar.com/sports/hockey/2014/04/12/50_years_later_maple_leafs_legend_bobby_baun_still_unstoppable.html.

5. Traina J. What Schilling's ankle looked like at infamous bloody sock game. November 12, 2014. http://www.foxsports.com/buzzer/story/curt-schilling-bloody-sock-ankle-photo-111214.

6. Rodrigues J. Manchester City football legend dies: Trautmann the impassable. *The Guardian.* July 19, 2013. http://www.theguardian.com/theguardian/from-the-archive-blog/2013/jul/19/bert-trautmann-manchester-city-fa-cup-1956.

QUICK ANSWERS TO COMMON QUESTIONS ABOUT SPORTS CONCUSSION

Q: If a concussion is suspected, who removes the youth athlete from practice or a game? A coach? A parent? An athletic trainer?

Dr. Kutcher: *Anyone in a position of responsibility, and that certainly includes all three. It can be difficult for parents to feel empowered to remove their child from participation. That said, if they have any concern about their child's safety, they absolutely have the right to do just that. I would stress, however, that working with the medical or coaching staff (or both) directly and in harmony is the preferred approach.*

Q: When the athlete has been taken out of play because of a suspected concussion and now is on the sideline, who does the evaluation? An athletic trainer? The school nurse or doctor? Or maybe a parent or coach?

Dr. Kutcher: *A medical evaluation of the athlete is best performed by a trained and licensed medical professional. Of course, not all medical professionals have the same level of training. If a physician is present and in a position of direct responsibility, she or he should obviously direct the evaluation. Athletic trainers are also trained specifically in recognizing concussion in the athletic environment. While non-medical professionals shouldn't be making diagnostic decisions, coaches and parents have a critical role to play in screening for injury if no medical personnel are present.*

Q: Should a school or league's concussion protocol have a defined return-to-play schedule?

Dr. Kutcher: *There should be a framework for the progression to returning to play in place, with clear milestones. Practically speaking, however, the exact timing of the process will depend on many factors, including the level of training and experience of those directing it. The basic principle, however, is that at each stage the patient should be given enough observation time for signs and symptoms to occur if they are going to.*

Q: While the concussion is healing, should schools make academic allowances for athletes in recovery?

Dr. Kutcher: *Absolutely. Although not every patient will require academic accommodations, they should always be considered. Much as with physical recovery, mental recovery requires time for rest and time for a gradual return to activity. And as with physical recovery, this process is best directed by a physician.*

Q: Who should give the final say for the athlete to resume practicing or playing?

Dr. Kutcher: *The return-to-play decision is a medical one. While the concussion itself may be a straightforward injury, there are many concurrent issues that require careful consideration. Additionally, no recovery should be treated as only a one- to two-week episode. The patient's prior medical history and future neurological health must also be considered. For these reasons, I stress that it is in the best interest of our patients that return-to-play decisions be made by a physician—preferably one with neurological training.*

Q: Is there a number of concussions that signals that an athlete should retire? Does the frequency of concussions matter?

Dr. Kutcher: *The number of concussions that have been diagnosed or suspected is only the beginning of the conversation about retirement. Certainly, the more injuries present, the higher the concern. That does not mean that any one number should trigger retirement. Every injury needs to be considered carefully and completely and then put into a bigger picture. Is there evidence of brain dysfunction that isn't resolving? What's happened between the concussions? Has the athlete had there any chronic issues such as headache or mood problems? How much overall contact has the athlete* experienced without getting concussed? All of these questions need to be answered.

At the same time, the frequency of concussions can be one of the clues that might lead to a recommendation of retirement. One possible explanation for frequent concussions is that the person has a low, or lowering, threshold for injury. Other explanations, however, may not be as concerning, such as a low threshold for producing symptoms, which might result in an athlete's receiving frequent concussion diagnoses with very little underlying injury. Some factors are modifiable and might make continued participation a reasonable choice if they are addressed, such as a dangerous style of play that can be adjusted through coaching or equipment concerns that can dealt with directly.

TERMS TO KNOW ABOUT CONCUSSIONS AND SPORTS

Baseline test: A test of brain function, usually given at the start of a season, to establish an athlete's normal memory function, balance, reaction time, and other variables. If an athlete is injured during the season, the test can be administered again and the new score can be compared with the original, baseline score to assess neurological processing and function.

Clinician: A general term referring to any individual who is licensed to practice and is practicing clinical medicine. Physicians are a subset of clinicians. Other types of clinicians who provide neurological care for patients include, but are not limited to, athletic trainers, physical therapists, and neuropsychologists.

Concussion: A traumatic brain injury caused by a blow or jolt to the head or neck. Concussions can range from mild to severe, and usually heal in a period of one to two weeks.

Migraine: A form of a headache sometimes triggered by concussion or post-concussive issues. Migraines typically involve sensitivity to light and sound, painful throbbing sensations, and vision issues. They can be chronic.

Neurologist: A physician who specializes in diagnosing and treating diseases of the nervous system and brain. Neurologists also treat brain injuries, such as concussion.

Neuropsychologist: A clinician who practices a mixture of psychology and neurology. Clinical neuropsychologists, who hold Ph.D. degrees, often work or consult with neurologists on evaluating patients and developing treatment plans.

Neurosurgeon: A physician who specializes in surgical treatment of brain, nerve, and spinal cord issues.

Physician: An individual who has graduated from medical school. A physician is either an M.D. (Medical Doctor) or a D.O. (Doctor of Osteopathy).

Post-concussive syndrome: A collection of neurological, psychiatric, or other symptoms that is present after a concussion is over.

Protocol: With respect to concussion, the set process that qualified medical professionals use to assess athletes. Most organized leagues and school systems have established concussion protocols to protect athlete health.

Return to play: A systematic process of gradually reintroducing a concussed athlete to activity. Effective return to play helps the brain readjust to athletic exertion.

Second-impact syndrome: A very rare but gravely serious condition arising when a concussed brain takes another blow. The second injury to the vulnerable brain can lead to brain swelling, resulting in serious disruption of brain function or even death.

Traumatic brain injury (TBI): An injury to the brain caused by its experiencing a force, for example, in an accident such as a car crash, fall, or athletic play. The force may come from a direct blow to the head (or helmet) or be the result of a hit to the body that causes a whiplash movement of the head and neck. A concussion is a form of TBI. Traumatic brain injuries vary in degree of seriousness.

RESOURCES TO LEARN MORE ABOUT SPORTS CONCUSSION

American Academy of Neurology's sports concussion toolkit:
www.aan.com/practice/sports-concussion-toolkit/

Virginia Tech's STAR helmet ratings:
http://www.beam.vt.edu/helmet/index.php

Dr. Kutcher's clinic:
TheSportsNeurologyClinic.com

Moms Team Youth Sports Concussion Safety Center:
www.momsteam.com/health-safety/concussion-safety

UCLA BrainSPORT—Dr. Christopher Giza:
https://www.uclahealth.org/brainsport/Pages/default.aspx

Concussion Legacy Foundation:
Concussionfoundation.org

Seeing Stars Foundation:
Seeingstarsfoundation.org

Center for Disease Control's HEADS UP Concussion in Youth Sports initiative:
http://www.cdc.gov/headsup/youthsports/

National Athletic Trainers Association (NATA) concussion resources:
http://www.nata.org/practice-patient-care/health-issues/concussion

Center for Disease Control's Sports Concussion Policies and Laws page:
http://www.cdc.gov/headsup/policy

Dr. Kutcher on Twitter: @JeffKutcherMD
Joanne C. Gerstner on Twitter: @JoanneCGerstner

ACKNOWLEDGMENTS

This project has been a nearly three-year labor of love for us, a remarkable shared journey of wanting to help athletes and those around them best understand the complex issue of concussion.

Sincere thanks to Dr. Christopher Giza, Spencer Helgren, Eric Hipple, Jason Hodges, Ellery Hollingsworth, Linherr Hollingsworth, Kristin Johnson, Kate Markgraf, Professor Andy Markovits, Andy Murray, Ben Utecht, and Pete Vaz for the time, openness, and generosity of spirit to share their stories and thoughts with us. Also a big "Thank you" to the American Academy of Neurology, the University of Michigan Athletic Department, the CORE Institute, the Sports

Neurology Clinic, graphic artist Stacey Fox, and the School of Journalism at Michigan State University for their support.

Our fantastic editors, especially Craig Panner and Emily Perry, and everybody at Oxford University Press have been great allies and resources in this project, who pushed us to a higher level.

We also must thank our families, loved ones, and friends for their encouragement and love. They went along on this ride too, and we are grateful.

We hope that this book helps bring some clarity to the discussion of concussions in youth sports. Both of us are sports fans and athletes since childhood. We want to see our culture become smarter about concussion at the same time that sports continue to be an important part of the human experience.

Jeff Kutcher, MD and Joanne C. Gerstner

INDEX

References to figures are denoted by an italicized *f*.